CRIME SIGNALS

ALSO BY DAVID GIVENS

Love Signals: A Practical Field Guide to the Body Language of Courtship

CRIME SIGNALS

HOW TO SPOT A CRIMINAL
BEFORE YOU BECOME A VICTIM

DAVID GIVENS, Ph.D.

ST. MARTIN'S PRESS ＊ NEW YORK

The names of some living individuals have been disguised to protect their identity. These names appear in quotes in this book.

www.stmartins.com

Design by Ruth Lee-Mui

Library of Congress Cataloging-in-Publication Data

Givens, David B.
  Crime signals : how to spot a criminal before you become a victim / David Givens.—1st ed.
     p. cm.
  Includes bibliographical references.
  ISBN-13: 978-0-312-36261-4
  ISBN-10: 0-312-36261-7
 1. Criminals—Study and teaching. 2. Body language. 3. Nonverbal communication.   I. Title.

HV6024.G58 2008
613.6'6—dc22

2007038866

First Edition: January 2008

10 9 8 7 6 5 4 3 2 1

For my mother, **Helen T. Givens,** with love

CONTENTS

ACKNOWLEDGMENTS

I would like to thank the following colleagues whose insights through the years helped shape this book: A. J. O. Anderson, John R. Atkins, Donald Brockington, Carol M. Eastman, Victor Goldkind, Henry T. Lewis, Foster W. Martin, Joe Navarro, Simon Ottenberg, Kenneth E. Read, Spencer L. Rogers, Thomas Sebeok, LaMont "Monty" West Jr., and David Willingham. I thank Yaniv Soha, my stellar young editor at St. Martin's Press, for his wisdom, grace, and guidance. Sincere thanks go to Eileen Cope, my agent at Trident Media Group in New York, for her support—and for making this project possible.

A PRELIMINARY MUSING

The whole thing is just a rotten shame.

—JULIE RIVETT, granddaughter of Dashiell
Hammett, commenting on the latest theft of the
Maltese Falcon

ON THE EVENING of December 5, 2006, I was in San Francisco at John's Grill—"Home of the Maltese Falcon"—having dinner with my research team. We'd spent the day in superior court, videotaping body language of judges and litigants in a study funded by the National Center for State Courts. Nobody, from bailiffs to judges to those on trial, seemed to mind our cameras.

After each taping, we spoke with the judge, plaintiff, and defendant—in separate debriefings—about how they'd read one another's courtroom demeanor that day. We showed them the videotapes and probed for insights on the role that body language had played in court. Our goal was to study how nonverbal communication worked alongside the official written transcript.

Sitting in historic John's Grill on Ellis Street, where Dashiell Hammett, author of *The Maltese Falcon* (1930), used to dine, I reflected on the voyeuristic nature of my craft. As an anthropologist, people watching is my game. From the size of a pupil within its iris to the gross anatomy of a shoulder shrug, I take careful notes on how bodies talk apart from words. If a dilated pupil shows excitement, a raised shoulder telegraphs an uncertain frame of mind. Both speak of moods not objectively revealed in speech. If detecting such cues requires that you become something of an obsessive observer, so be it.

Crime Signals reports my own observations of criminal body language, and shares the wisdom of judges, jurors, journalists, police, and offenders themselves. We explore body talk in big cases, like those of Scott Peterson and Martha Stewart, and in the wee ones covered by hometown papers. All of the criminal convictions and suspects reported in *Crime Signals* are real, factual, and available on the public record. Without belittling or blaming perpetrators, we decode their visible body language for clues. What we find could help safeguard you from the evil effects of crime.

Unfortunately, crime is never ending. On February 10, 2007, John Konstin, owner of John's Grill, noticed that his restaurant's prized replica of the Maltese Falcon was missing from its locked display case. In Hammett's novel, the original figurine, proffered as a gift from the island of Malta in 1539 to King Charles V of Spain, had been lost or stolen several times. Pirates made off with the statuette, which eventually found its way to Paris.

Finally, private eye Sam Spade was hired to find the missing bird, several plaster replicas of which were later made for the 1941 film version of Hammett's book. In *The Maltese Falcon*, Humphrey Bogart played the starring role of Sam Spade, and years later, in 1995, John's Grill was given one of the movie replicas of the figurine to display in its Hammett museum upstairs.

The heist was, as Hammett's granddaughter described it, "a rotten shame." If Sam Spade were around today, his keen eye for detail would surely be indispensable in solving the latest case of the missing Maltese Falcon. I trust that as he investigated, he would watch body language—very carefully—for crime signals.

CRIME SIGNALS

CRIME SIGNALS
BEFORE AND AFTER THE CRIME

I can never bring you to realize the importance of sleeves, the suggestiveness of thumbnails, or the great issues that may hang from a bootlace.

—SHERLOCK HOLMES,
to Watson, in "A Case of Identity"

AS SHERLOCK HOLMES wisely taught, a crime seldom happens in a vacuum. Crimes rarely go unannounced, without prior notice, clues, or warnings. Before and after the swindle, stabbing, jewel theft, sexual assault, or mysterious death by poisoning there are clearly readable signs. Seeing an armed robber shake a pistol in your face is an obvious and tangible sign of danger. The most commonly experienced danger signs, however, are intangible feelings and suppositions that *something is wrong*.

The highly publicized murder of Kristin Lardner, twenty-one, is a case in point. Her homicidal boyfriend, Michael Cartier, twenty-two, telegraphed a medley of tangible and intangible warning signs before he killed Kristin on a Boston sidewalk with his .38. Had Kristin heeded Michael's danger signs, she might be alive today.

"I had a very bad feeling about him when I met him," Kristin Lardner's friend Lisa recalled (Lardner 1995, 155). But blinded by love, Kristin herself felt good about Michael, and described the tall, black-haired, blue-eyed nightclub bouncer as "cute." That he wore a large tattoo of a castle drawn prominently on his neck did not seem to matter. As we will see, tattoos worn on the face, forehead, or neck—called "radical tattoos" or "job stoppers" in the tattooing business—can often raise serious crime issues. Tattoos worn on or about the face can scream, "I'm in your face!"

For Michael Cartier, the neck tattoo forewarned of antisocial personality disorder or APD. When they first met, in February 1992, Michael was friendly, charming, and sweet. He took Kristin to dinner and escorted her to clubs. For Valentine's Day, he gave her a rose and a teddy bear. Michael swept the promising young art student off her feet with devoted affection until early in March 1992, when he screamed in anger, punched Kristin's bedroom wall, and then savagely punched Kristin in the head (Lardner 1995, 161). Barely a month had passed before the tattoo's tragic promise of cruelty came true.

In April 1992, Michael's anger shifted into chronic mode. On April 15, he argued with Kristin and shoved her down on a sidewalk near the Boston University campus. When she got up, he tossed stones at her and struck her in the calf with a hurled steel rod. Michael threw her on the sidewalk again, cursed her, then threw Kristin into the street and brutally kicked her legs and head. Around two o'clock the next morning, April 16, concerned motorists stopped to help Kristin home.

If these were incredibly tangible danger signs, there were others Michael tried to hide. He had a three-page criminal record and had spent time in jail. In 1989 at a Massachusetts café, he injected his own blood from a syringe into a ketchup bottle as his skinhead friends watched and laughed (Lardner 1995, 102). In 1990, he beat his previous girlfriend, Rose Ryan, and savagely attacked her with a pair of scissors.

Like Kristin's, Rose Ryan's romance with Michael ended after lasting barely a month. Rose and Michael were out walking in the Boston Common when, without warning, he playfully threw her into a city trash can. Playful or not, his behavior clearly showed that "something was wrong." They argued afterward, and then, as she explained, "Something stung the side of my head. It came unexpectedly, like a bird's dropping. He had punched me. Bare knuckles, backed by his full weight" (Ryan 1993).

I call Michael Cartier's nonverbal warning signs "crime signals." Had Kristin Lardner only known the history and breadth of her boyfriend's crime signals, she might have moved from Boston to a safer place far away. But, trusting her fate to police protection, she sought a restraining order instead. Then on May 30, 1992—after Kristin left her boyfriend, after she received her court-mandated restraining order, after weeks of relentless stalking by her predatory ex-boyfriend—Michael Cartier approached Kristin from behind and shot her in the back of the head with his pistol. After she'd fallen, mortally wounded, to the sidewalk, he shot her twice more. An hour later, Michael Cartier was found dead in his own apartment after killing himself with the same .38.

"SOMETHING IS WRONG"

Crime is an act committed or omitted in violation of a law. *Crime Signals* investigates the body language of perpetrators before and after the crime. What nonverbal warning signs should you look for to protect yourself and your loved ones from harm?

"He lived upstairs, but he always seemed creepy." This

according to the woman who, after seeing his mug shot on *The Oprah Winfrey Show*, turned her fugitive neighbor in to the FBI. But what does "creepy" mean? In the pages that follow, I'll break "creepy" into easy-to-identify nonverbal cues. As an anthropologist and specialist in nonverbal communication, I have taught police officers, FBI agents, and members of the intelligence community to search beneath words for behavioral clues that spell danger. Knowing what to look for makes the world feel safer.

What Sherlock Holmes did for the crime novel, *Crime Signals* does for the real world of crime. Before writing his Sherlock Holmes mysteries, Arthur Conan Doyle was a practicing physician. Doyle's fascination with clues grew from his earlier study of disease symptoms. Both are signals that "something is wrong."

Combining the keen eye of Sherlock Holmes with the latest discoveries in forensic science, nonverbal studies, and behavioral neurology, *Crime Signals* explores the most telling cues of evil intent. From a stranger's uninvited stare on the subway to unfamiliar footsteps outside your door, body language enables you to discern crimes in the making before they occur. Should a crime take place, body language can lead you through the confusing verbiage of alibis to unspoken, sometimes unspeakable truths.

WHAT ARE CRIME SIGNALS?

Crime signals are perceptible signs disclosing that someone has broken, or is about to break, the law. Like behavioral red flags, crime signals show that something bad is about to happen, or already has. Criminals seldom verbalize their evil intentions beforehand. To the victim, treachery is more likely to be revealed in body movements and demeanor than in vocal comments. In the criminal world, nonverbal signs, signals, and cues speak louder than words.

Murderers, sexual predators, terrorists, and thieves all emit telling cues before their misdeeds. A terrorist's intent can show in his eyes. When U.S. Transportation Security Administration analyst Carl Maccario reviewed videotapes of the September 11, 2001, hijackers going through security at Dulles International Airport, he noticed that all three men withheld their gaze from the security guards: "They all looked away and had their heads down," he said (Frank 2005a).

For police officers, gaze avoidance can be a divulging cue. When occupants of a vehicle avoid looking at the patrol car cruising beside them, they could have something to hide. As an officer explained, looking away makes them think, in their own minds, that they somehow "disappear." For police on patrol, gaze aversion counts as one of the top five street signs of suspicion.

Avoiding eye contact with authorities is a normal human response. Called "cutoff" by anthropologist Adam Kendon, visual avoidance is rooted in primate biology. Subordinate gorillas, for instance, typically avert their eyes from a dominant silverback's threatening stare. They look away to avoid contact.

Among human beings, gaze avoidance begins early in childhood. Facing away from a stranger's eyes reduces a baby's blood pressure and slows its heartbeat rate. Babies handle the stress of visual encounters with potentially threatening adults by turning their eyes downward or away to the side. Older children playfully cover their eyes with their hands to disappear from view, as if to say, "You can't see me now!"

In effect, the drilled and disciplined September 11 terrorists behaved like children. All three on the video bent their heads down and looked away. Without practice or rehearsal beforehand, the trio simultaneously displayed the identical crime signal. Had security guards recognized cutoff as a cue, as the TSA's Maccario did months after the hijacking, they might have stopped the men to ask probing questions. September 11, 2001, might have remained just an ordinary day.

ANOMALOUS CRIME SIGNALS

When the U.S. threat level rises, citizens are warned to be cautious: "Be alert to suspicious activity and report it." But what is suspicious? As I'll show you throughout this book, suspicious behavior is really *anomalous* behavior. Anomalous behavior is that which deviates from the norm, and a great many crime signals are intrinsically unusual—perceptibly abnormal.

Here's an example. In December 2005, a seventy-five-year-old woman stopped to visit her elderly mother at Overlake Hospital Medical Center in Bellevue, Washington. She rode up the elevator with three well-dressed men in their midthirties. Suddenly, it appeared that one of the men had his foot caught in the closing door. He asked the woman for assistance, and as she bent down to help free his trapped shoe, an accomplice reached his hand into her purse and seized her wallet. When the doors opened, the three men physically ushered her out of the elevator and stayed inside as the doors closed. Moments later, safely inside her mother's hospital room, the good Samaritan discovered her wallet was missing.

"I thought I was in a safe place," she told police (Bach 2005). Safe? Usually, but on that day an anomalous crime signal had been sent. A man bent forward in the elevator trying to free his shoe. How often do feet get caught in elevators? Few of us will ever witness such an aberrant event. Figures compiled in "The Elevator World Vertical Transportation Industry Profile" put the chances of getting hurt in an elevator at one in twelve million.

Clearly, the behavior seen by the lady from Bellevue was unusual—and should therefore have been suspicious.

After September 11, 2001, software was developed to detect such anomalous behaviors in airport elevators. Captured on closed-circuit cameras, nonverbal actions today are coded by computers as being either normal or abnormal. Staying too long in an elevator, for instance, is classified as abnormal. The dawdling would set off a remote alarm to notify airport security. Abnormal physical movements in the elevator—a man assembling a mechanism or stooping to open a suitcase on the floor—would do the same.

> **Captured on closed-circuit cameras, nonverbal actions are coded by computers as being either normal or abnormal.**

The improbable elevator scene in Bellevue—a man stooped over to free his "trapped" foot—should have sounded a mental alarm. Statistically, the behavior was aberrant. Crime signals flashed a red warning: "Strange behavior! Watch your purse!"

Since life is predictable most of the time, anomalies are telling:

- A man in a shopping mall stoops under a heavy backpack (bomb materials can weigh twenty-two to twenty-six pounds).
- At your supermarket, five men in a vehicle park in a handicapped space near the store's entrance.
- Motionless customers stand like statues inside a convenience store (an armed robbery is under way).
- On a warm July day, two men in bulky jackets run down a sidewalk filled with walkers.

- Four men peer into a liquor store. Each wears at least one conspicuous red item of clothing (see chapter 8, "Reading the Gang Signs").
- A man in jogging clothes smokes a cigarette and stretches beside his parked van. Preparing to "jog," he keeps a steady eye on comings and goings at the nearby bank.
- Three men you've never seen before enter your favorite diner (chance?); later, the same men loiter outside your office building (coincidence?); after work, they board your commuter train (alarm bell!).

THE NONVERBAL WORLD OF CRIME

Staying alert to crime signals helps keep you safer, and helps you protect your loved ones. Fortunately, most animals, including human beings, give advance warning before they attack. Before biting, a frilled lizard rears up and erects its neck frill to bluff. Before actually striking, a cobra vertically rears and spreads its hood. Before charging, a bull takes several stiff steps forward and turns sideways to show you the widest, most threatening part of its body. To bluff before attacking, the bull looms large.

Before offending, pedophiles groom their victims with unusual attention, favors, and gifts. Before killing, stalkers follow their victims for days, show up uninvited in victims' homes, and give inappropriate gifts. Street gangs declare themselves with tattoos, unusual hand gestures, and color-coded clothing. For those who pay attention, crime signals are forewarnings: Something wicked this way comes. We may read them or weep.

Before we begin our fieldwork in Crimeland, I should explain my lifelong fascination with nonverbal communication and body language. For as long as I can remember, I've been a committed people watcher. I had little idea what prompted my interest, though, until college. There, as an anthropology student at the

University of Washington in Seattle, I learned that the postures, body movements, and facial expressions that enthralled me were more than mere gestures; they were *signals*.

From the Latin word *signalis*, for "sign," a signal is an indicator that serves as a means of communication (Soukhanov 1992, 1678). It was not the gestures that had caught my fancy, but what the gestures conveyed. In short, my fascination had been with the voiceless emotions, hidden intentions, and secret agendas revealed in body talk. What mattered to me most was the speechless dialogue that went on beneath people's words. As you're about to see, nowhere does speechless dialogue matter more than in the verbally deceptive world of crime.

As an anthropologist who studies body language, I see crime through a different lens from the forensic eyepiece of criminologists, judges, lawyers, and police. Academic articles, court records, law books, and police files consist mainly of words. What I look for in lawbreakers are gestures, body movements, physical actions, and demeanor. Whereas police ask questions, lawyers depose, and judges take notes, I watch eyes, lips, shoulders, and hands. Should a defendant suddenly drop his eyes, tighten his mouth, shrug his shoulders, or roll up a palm, I take note. As Sherlock Holmes taught, there is uncommon meaning in the commonplace.

You are cordially invited on a nonverbal tour of the crime world. Look but do not touch. The denizens of this world can be dangerous. As the Australian crocodile hunter, Steve Irwin, used to say of his ill-tempered crocs, "Danger, danger!" Human beings, we will see, are far more dangerous than crocodiles. To begin our fieldwork, let's examine the crime signals of some of the most insidious—and common—offenders. What do their bodies say when they lie?

1

THE LOOK OF A LIE

I did not have sexual relations with that woman, Miss Lewinsky.

—WILLIAM JEFFERSON CLINTON

CONTEXT IS EVERYTHING in body language. A pointed index finger can mean one thing in an art museum, and something else entirely at a congressional hearing. Aimed at a Renoir in the Louvre, a pointed forefinger can refer to the painting as if to say, "Look." Aimed at a congressional panel, the same stiffened finger can say, "I'm lying."

The pointed index finger of deceit was seen by millions who watched Baltimore Orioles first baseman Rafael Palmeiro testify before a U.S. congressional hearing on March 17, 2005. In his opening statement, Palmeiro aggressively stabbed his index finger at members of the panel and said, "I have never used steroids. Period. I don't know how to say it any more clearly than that. Never" (Dodd and Bodley 2005).

Refusing to testify until subpoenaed, Palmeiro later claimed his finger point was spontaneous. "I was just speaking from the heart, man," he explained. Nearly six months later, on August 1, 2005, after testing positive for the drug stanozolol, Palmeiro received a ten-day suspension for violating baseball's steroid policy. U.S. representative John Sweeney of New York accused Palmeiro of "audacious lying."

By pointing his finger, Rafael Palmeiro gave what many saw as an overly dramatic response to the accusation of steroid abuse. To quote the famous line from Shakespeare's *Hamlet*, "Me thinks he protest too much."

BODIES DO NOT LIE

Lawbreakers lie to cover up their offenses. Since they must lie to survive, offenders are generally skilled at deception and often sound convincing. But while the tongue tells a lie, the body cannot. As you listen to words, look to the body—especially to hands, shoulders, lips, and eyes—for truth.

A lie is a statement deliberately meant to give a wrong impression or to deceive. The English word "lie" comes from the seven-thousand-year-old Indo-European root *leugh-*, "to tell a lie." Fundamentally about secrecy and concealing, deceit is an ancient human practice with deep roots in animal psychology.

Deceit is truly widespread in the animal kingdom. Non-poisonous flies and snakes adopt warning marks and coloration of poisonous species to seem more harmful than they are. The ability to deceive is highly evolved in primates. Our closest primate relative, the chimpanzee, is an especially gifted deceiver.

Zoologist Frans de Waal observed a young male, Dandy, who deliberately withheld cues of excitement to deceive other chimps about the location of hidden grapefruit. Dandy later consumed all the grapefruit by himself. Primatologist Jane Goodall watched as Figan, a nine-year-old male, deliberately withheld food calls to conceal a bunch of ripe bananas. Figan later consumed all the bananas by himself.

Like chimpanzees, people withhold information for their own profit or gain. When asked about their unscrupulous actions, people, unlike chimps, become *verbally* deceptive. Many undermine their vocal lies, however, with the same excessively emotional, overwrought hand gesture given by Rafael Palmeiro. In the context of a verbal lie, the index finger point is singularly revealing and should prompt you to question whether the speaker's words are true.

Seven years before Palmeiro made his public point, you may have witnessed the most infamous finger-pointing display ever seen on national or international TV. On January 26, 1998, President William Jefferson Clinton pointed aggressively at the American people and said, "I did not have sexual relations with that woman, Miss Lewinsky." Seven months later, sitting in the Map Room of the White House on August 17, Clinton made a televised statement to the American people: "Indeed, I did have a relationship with Miss Lewinsky that was not appropriate." On January 14, 1999, Clinton faced impeachment over the affair on charges of perjury and obstruction of justice.

"He doth protest too much" goes for Clinton as well as for Palmeiro. Both men's index fingers fervently extended to show indignation—self-righteous anger—at those who accused them of wrongdoing. Nonverbally, however, there was less truth in their statements than raw anger. The truth was not in the words but in the act of pointing.

THE SHOE BOMBER'S POINT

Around the world, stabbing motions of the index finger are given in wrath and ire. A classic case of indignant pointing belongs to self-described al Qaeda terrorist Richard Reid. Reid was convicted on January 30, 2003, of trying to blow up an American Airlines Paris-to-Miami flight with a bomb hidden in his shoe. Just before he was handcuffed in court, Reid leaned forward, pointed at the judge, and yelled anti-American sentiments. Earlier, Reid's suspicious behavior—bending down to ignite his shoe bomb's fuse with a lighted match—had caught the attention of passengers and flight crew, who quickly subdued him. Reid is the reason airports x-ray footwear today.

Pointing a stiffened index finger at another person is a widespread human sign of aggression—not of truth. The pointing gesture is assisted by an extra forearm muscle, extensor indicis, which evolved explicitly to assist the index finger's point. Incited by palpably negative emotions, pointing at another is almost universally deemed to be an unfriendly, rude, and even hostile act. It's no wonder, then, that while casting spells, tribal sorcerers aim their evil energies by pointing at victims with wands or extended forefingers.

INDIGNANT LYING: THE CASE OF THE MISSING DIGIT

Criminals often cover up their lies with aggressive displays of anger. Lips snarl, brows lower, eyes glare, and voices snap as they mouth words that are mostly untrue. Not only do anger signs deflect attention away from lies, they also warn listeners away from questioning the liar. Like growling dogs, angry liars threaten to bite.

On March 22, 2005, thirty-nine-year-old Anna Ayala found a one-and-a-half-inch-long dismembered human finger in her bowl of chili at a San Jose, California, Wendy's. The well-manicured fingertip entered Ayala's mouth when she took a bite. It was "kind of hard, crunchy," she said. Anna reported the incident to Wendy's staff, and in the process unleashed a nationwide scandal that cost Wendy's millions of dollars in business as customers avoided its fast-food stores.

"There's no words to describe what I felt. It's sick, it's disgusting," Ayala said. Shortly after the incident, she filed a claim accusing Wendy's of negligent food handling. But under intense scrutiny as investigators closed in, she later withdrew the claim and sought seclusion in her Las Vegas home. Meanwhile, Wendy's and police continued to pursue the case. Authorities searched a fingerprint database to learn who the finger belonged to, but were unsuccessful, and testing was done to learn if the digit was raw or cooked.

Investigators found no fault with Wendy's or its suppliers, and suspicion turned to Ayala herself. In an interview at her home with CBS news reporter Joe Vasquez on April 8, 2005, Ayala answered the reporter's questions with repeated displays of verbal and nonverbal anger.

"Anna, did you plant the finger?" Vasquez had asked.

"She paused," Vasquez reported in his story. "And she shot me an 'if looks could kill' stare. 'Where would I get a damn finger, for God sakes!?' "

SIGNS OF ANGER

Anger is a usually unpleasant feeling of annoyance, resentment, or rage. It is a mammalian elaboration of earlier reptilian behaviors designed for fighting and displaying dominance, and it shows itself in frowning, jaws tensed for biting, palm-down overhand-beating gestures, tense or tightened lips, pointed fingers, a growling voice, and glaring. Studies suggest that anger shows most prominently in the lower face and in contortions around one's frowning eyebrows. Corrugator muscles, blended with frontalis and orbicularis oculi muscles, draw eyebrows downward as if to shield the eyes, producing vertical furrows above the nose. The anger signs originally reported by Charles Darwin in 1872—body held erect, contracted brows, compressed mouth, flared nostrils, and "flashing eyes"—are expressly the same today.

Anna Ayala's angry answer neither intimidated nor deflected Joe Vasquez.

"Anna, for the record, you did not put any finger in any chili?"

" 'No!' she snapped back with a bite in her voice. 'That is the stupidest thing that they can say. Now, I'm very angry' " (Vasquez 2005).

As with Bill Clinton and Rafael Palmeiro, there was less truth in Anna Ayala's statements than emotional anger. On January 18, 2006, Ayala was sentenced to nine years in prison for conspiracy to file a false insurance claim and attempted grand theft from Wendy's. Her husband, Jaime Plascencia, forty-four, who'd bought the severed finger from a coworker in the first place, was sentenced to twelve years and four months.

NONVERBAL LOCKDOWN: THE SCOTT PETERSON CASE

Like Clinton and Palmeiro, some people point while lying, but not all pointers lie. In fact, for a minority of offenders, deception shows in the complete absence of gestures. Nonverbal lockdown—no body language at all—can reveal as much about the absence of an emotion as indignant pointing can reveal about its presence. Since sociopathic lawbreakers don't experience normal feelings of guilt or remorse, they show fewer nonverbal signs of emotion when they lie. In short, they protest too little.

For some offenders, deception is disclosed by a complete absence of gestures.

No pointed finger was given by Scott Peterson, for example. On November 12, 2004, in Redwood City, California, Peterson was convicted for the first-degree murder of his wife, Laci, and the second-degree murder of their unborn son, Conner. In court, Scott showed no bodily signs of indignation—or any other feeling, for that matter—save the muted, intellectual emotion psychologists call "interest." Indeed, as jurors voiced their final decisions, one by one, to convict him, Peterson gazed at each with a completely expressionless face. Reportedly, none of the jurors met his eyes.

To lie by omission is to withhold relevant information by remaining silent. As a sign of deception, a composed demeanor and deadpan face can be as telling as Clinton's and Palmeiro's pointing digits. Again, showing no indignation whatsoever suggests the absence of emotion, much as demonstrative hand gestures can reveal its presence. After his murder trial, jurors commented that Peterson had seemed apathetic, indifferent, and unemotional in court throughout the six-month ordeal.

MISREADING SCOTT PETERSON'S MOUTH

If you look carefully at Scott Peterson's mouth in its reposed state, you will notice that his lips curve slightly upward at the outer corners. When he smiles, they angle up higher still. Many who saw him on TV misread

Peterson's face as smirking of superiority and disdain. At rest, however, it was just an expressionless face. Studies show that we tend to read emotion into the features of a deadpan face when it's not really there.

In Peterson's case, deception was visible months before his trial. On Christmas Eve 2002, Laci's mother, Sharon Rocha, drove to her daughter's home immediately after Scott reported Laci missing. Police were already on the scene. When Scott arrived, Laci's mom observed that he "didn't look very upset and certainly not panicked" (Rocha 2006, 58). Later, she saw Scott standing alone in his driveway staring into the distance with a "strangely blank look on his face" (Rocha 2006, 58). Feeling sorry for Scott at the time, Sharon Rocha stepped forward to comfort him with a hug. As she moved toward Scott, he angled his body and shoulders away to his left. When she tried a second time to hug him, Scott again angled leftward to avoid her embrace.

Though he spoke to her in the driveway, Scott wouldn't make eye contact with his own mother-in-law, who was simply offering maternal comfort in the storm. What for her was an emotional storm was for him, apparently, just a breeze.

Angling away to one's right or left is a form of cutoff anthropologists call "angular distance." Angular distance is the spatial orientation, measured in degrees, of a listener's upper body in relation to a speaker's, either facing or angling away. Greater angular distance—turning farther away to the right or left—substitutes for greater linear distance, and reveals how we truly feel about someone.

Our upper body unwittingly squares up to, addresses, and "aims" at those we confide in and trust, but twists away from disliked persons and those we mistrust. Scott's amplified angular distance that evening clearly showed he had something to hide. Sharon Rocha didn't need an anthropologist to advise that Scott's "something" was terribly, terribly wrong.

"I'M NOT A CROOK"

Known to be ill at ease around people, former President Richard Milhous Nixon revealed his discomfort with exaggerated angular distance to "remove" himself from those nearby. White House photographs taken at staff meetings in the early 1970s show a seated Mr. Nixon with shoulders turned and twisted completely away from his advisers at angles of ninety degrees. On November 17, 1973, nine months before he literally removed himself from his own presidency, a tense Mr. Nixon maintained his innocence in the Watergate burglary case by stating, "I'm not a crook." In his political career, the physical demeanor of "Tricky Dick," as detractors called him, stood visibly at odds with his spoken words.

Throughout the investigation of Laci Peterson's disappearance, Scott Peterson showed few indications of grief or sadness. He displayed no shock, remorse, surprise, disgust, or anger. Scott did not blink faster, his lips did not tighten, his eyebrows did not lift. His body withdrew in full-fledged nonverbal lockdown. As a relative noted, Scott got more upset over a piece of burned barbecued chicken than over his missing wife.

Since Peterson never testified, we did not see his demeanor under oath on the witness stand. But between his wife's disappearance and his own arrest, he made several TV appearances and put his body squarely on prime-time display. Nonverbally, the most telling show was his January 27, 2003, *Good Morning America* interview with Diane Sawyer.

At the beginning of the interview, Scott cried as he told of walking their golden retriever, McKenzie, in the park where his wife used to walk the dog. But Scott's rare show of emotion stood in stark contrast to his cold demeanor in subsequent interviews, and later in court. In the *Good Morning America* segment, a window opened on Peterson's deceptive body language:

"Did you murder your wife?" Sawyer had asked point-blank.

"No," Scott answered. His demeanor was visibly subdued, and his tone of voice calm. Dressed in a white shirt, mauve tie, and tan suit with a "Missing Laci" button on its left lapel, Peterson comported himself as a clean-cut, eager young man on a job interview. He smiled, leaned forward, tilted his head sideward, coyly clasped his hands together in his lap, and innocently gazed into Sawyer's eyes.

Peterson looked as charming on TV as he'd looked to Sharon Rocha at their first meeting in Morro Bay, California, outside the Pacific Café. But immediately after his televised denial to Sawyer— "No"—Scott hemmed and hawed, punctuated his monotone answers with "uhs," "ahs," and "ums," and made numerous hesitations with audible, breathy exhalations. Vocally, by almost any standard of paralanguage, Peterson's repeated pauses test positive for deception.

Vocal tension, throat tightness, and throat clearings are highly responsive to stimuli from the emotional brain. The slightest anxiety can tighten a voice box. Neural impulses are carried by special visceral nerves, originally designed for feeding, which are unusually sensitive to transitory sentiments, feelings, and moods. While lying, gut feelings of anxiety and nervousness showed as Scott's throat, larynx, and pharynx muscles tightened. As Scott's tongue pronounced the words, his throat gave voice to his lies.

FROM *AMERICA'S DUMBEST CRIMINALS*

Responding to a home burglary in Brunswick, Georgia, police officers asked the victim if anything was missing from his home. He answered that someone had stolen his marijuana. When officers asked him to
repeat what they'd just heard, the victim's eyes widened.

"Are you admitting to possessing marijuana?" they asked.

"I . . . uh . . . well, no . . . not really," he stammered, adding, "Well . . . nothing, uh . . . I . . . oh, never mind" (Butler et al. 2000, 10). Since there was no
marijuana in his home, the police left and shared a good laugh.

Later in her interview, Sawyer asked Peterson if he'd told police about his affair with girlfriend Amber Frey: "Did you tell the
police?"

"I told the police immediately," Scott answered. But according
to the case's lead detective, Craig Grogan, Scott's answer was a
bald-faced lie. Grogan's observation that the defendant had verbally
lied corroborated the nonverbal evidence in Sawyer's interview—
Scott's hemming, hawing, and uh-filled pauses, each of which
pointed to deception.

Later, when the *Good Morning America* segment was shown
in court, jurors got to see Scott Peterson's body language in tandem with his words. For a nonverbal analysis, this is the best of
all possible worlds. Jurors could see Peterson's body language in
different contexts, and presented with a variety of topics. The
defendant could lie about one thing, tell the truth about another, and abstain on yet another. In a long interview, differences and similarities in contextual demeanor can be telling.

"Did you murder your wife?" "Did you tell the police?" Scott
answered both questions using precisely the same body language.

For each, he was quietly collected and composed. There were no exclamatory voice tones, no adamant hand gestures, no insistent head shakes of denial. He lied in both answers, so his nonverbal demeanor was predictably the same. Save for a labored larynx, on the video Scott seemed unruffled and relaxed.

One of the jurors, however, was not so relaxed. As he watched Scott answer Sawyer's second question—"Did you tell the police?"—Juror 8 "rolled his eyes, shook his head and stared at Peterson in apparent disbelief" (Hewitt et al. 2004, 71). Scott's demeanor while answering Diane's first question—"Did you murder your wife?"—was suspiciously like that while answering the second: seemingly calm and collected.

Upon conviction, Scott Peterson showed no emotion, save for a visibly clenched jaw, according to eyewitness Tim Ryan, a CBS Radio News reporter in the courtroom. The jaw clench, usually a sign of anger, is given as masseter muscles tense the jaws in preparation for biting. The trigeminal nerve (cranial V), which contracts these muscles, is an emotionally sensitive, special visceral nerve. For a fleeting moment, at least, Scott's face tipped his hand.

Jurors in the case suggested that Peterson's lack of visible emotion is what led to his death sentence. Juror Michael Belmessieri complained that Scott showed "no remorse." Juror Greg Beratlis would have liked to hear the sound of Peterson's voice on the witness stand. For juror Richelle Nice, Scott's show of "no emotion" upon hearing the verdict spoke "a thousand words." For all the thousands of words actually spoken in court, the single most memorable image was the defendant's neutral, expressionless, deadpan face. In speech and demeanor, he was emphatically, nonverbally guilty.

RESEARCH ON NONVERBAL SIGNS OF LYING

In "A Case of Identity," Sherlock Holmes observes a suspect's stammering speech, his "head sunk upon his breast," and the "glitter of moisture on his brow." Though Miss Sutherland's evil stepfather never confesses to masking his face and disguising his voice to woo her affection, his body gives voice to the lie. "There's a cold-blooded scoundrel!" Holmes concludes.

In 1887, Arthur Conan Doyle had Holmes interpret perspiration as a sign of deception. He did so thirty-four years before the polygraph test was invented in 1921. A polygraph measures physiological arousal as signaled by changes in sweating, blood pressure, breathing rate, and pulse. Today it is well established that the excretion of eccrine-gland moisture—sweat—onto the palmar surface of the hands occurs in response to anxiety, stress, and fear.

Our bodies rely on movement to deliver moisture to the skin's surface. Myoepithelial cells, which contain smooth, visceral-muscle-like organs, contract to squeeze the sweaty fluid through thin ducts in the skin. The tiny cells, which are linked to sympathetic—"fight-or-flight"—nerve fibers, also contract in response to adrenaline.

The best place to see nervous sweat is not on the brow itself but on the skin above one's upper lip. Tiny beads of sweat appear there first and then become visible on the forehead and temples. Sweating is a sign that the sympathetic nervous system has been aroused by the brain's fear center, the almond-shaped amygdala. Of course, it's up to the observer to explain what caused the sudden arousal. Could it be due to the fear of being disbelieved, or the fear of actually telling a lie? Seeing moisture on an upper lip in the midst of verbal denial likely suggests the latter.

A long-standing goal of research into the nonverbal has been to find reliable signs of deception. The quest is fueled by popular and scientific observations that deceit is oftentimes accompanied by unconscious signs of anxiety, stress, or shame.

Laboratory studies show that certain signals used while speaking—such as gaze aversion downward or a decreased rate of head and hand movements—do accompany lies. At the least, deception cues provide probing points that can guide inquiry regarding possible lies, much as galvanic skin response, breathing tempo, and heart rate measure autonomic stress in the polygraph.

Whatever the method, analysts have one thing in common: they do not see the lie directly, but by means of body language. Both reflect autonomic-nervous-system arousal, not actual lying. Between the arousal—disclosed by pointed finger or rapid pulse—and the lie is a vast interpretive chasm. An analyst's job is to bridge the explanation gap through a mixture of art and science.

In their article "Individual Differences in Hand Movements During Deception," social psychologist Aldert Vrij and his colleagues observe that people make "fewer hand movements during deception compared to truth-telling" (Vrij et al. 1997, 97). From his own analyses of videotaped interrogations, Joe Navarro, former FBI special agent, observed that deceivers are less likely than truth tellers to use what he calls "gravity-defying" gestures—such as raising the eyebrows, lifting the toes while seated, and rising up on the toes while standing—to add emphasis at the end of their sentences.

While speaking, a lower rate of head nodding, a higher blinking rate, and use of fewer hand gestures are likely to signal deception.

Since antigravity signs mark conviction, deceivers rarely use them. Emotionally, they behave as if they had little faith in their own words. Lack of conviction explains Scott Peterson's mumbling and anemic voice. According to Nick Flint of the Behavioral Analysis Training Institute in Santa Rosa, California, there are intellectual reasons for lack of self-confidence while telling lies. Making up verbal details to flesh out a lie takes more mental energy than remembering readily available true details. When Scott Peterson was not telling the truth, Flint noted, he lowered the volume of his voice (CBS 2004). With less cognitive investment, the body has a harder time standing behind that which is merely imagined, so body language appears less insistent and convincing.

True-life studies of lying are, unfortunately, few and far between. Based on unrealistic experiments with ambiguous study designs, the hundreds of laboratory studies of lie-detecting ability shed little light on the issue. Usually, college students are asked to play roles as fictitious liars in experiments designed to see if fellow-student judges can spot the lie. Missing in such artificial performances, of course, are the serious consequences of lying to real-life police officers, judges, and juries. However, in one ingenious study that combined elements of realistic deception with lab lying, University of San Francisco psychologists Paul Ekman and Maureen O'Sullivan discovered what they call "ultimate wizards."

Ultimate wizards are a very select group of people who, from nonverbal cues and word usage, can consistently detect deception. These human lie detectors stand head and shoulders above average study subjects. Exceptional observation skills are what help the intuitive wizards see what others miss. While most subjects score little better than chance—in the 50 percent range, getting half right and half wrong—wizards are right more than 80 percent of the time.

With training in body language—learning to decipher several nonverbal cues simultaneously—you, too, can attain wizardly status. Here's a list of cues that someone may not be telling you the whole truth:

· Indignant pointing with a stiffened index finger
· Glaring, "if looks could kill" anger
· Nonverbal lockdown: complete absence of gestures
· Facing and angling away: angular distance
· Vocal tension, throat tightness, throat clearings
· Acute episodes of stammering, hemming, and hawing
· Showing no emotion
· Telling moisture above the upper lip

In the next chapter, you will learn how to read deception from four of the body's most telling parts: hands, shoulders, lips, and eyes. For protection against an array of criminals, you should know what these emotional body parts have to say.

2

THE MEANING IN HANDS, SHOULDERS, LIPS, AND EYES

Once you've been a cop, you never look at people the same. . . .
You read their clothes, their hair, most of all their eyes.

—MARK FUHRMAN

IN HER BOOK *Louder Than Words*, Marjorie Vargas writes, "As a child, I never could understand how my mother knew every time I told her a lie" (Vargas 1986, 12). Mother knew, of course, because when children lie, their whole bodies participate in the deception. I call this naive, unedited physical response while lying a "whole-body lie."

"Did you eat your sister's candy?" Should the guilty child answer, "No," you will see her ears redden, head tilt sideward, eyebrows lift, eyes widen, eyeballs drop, lips pout, shoulders shrug, body angle away, hands clasp at the body's midline, and feet rotate inward to a pigeon-toed posture. Seeing these signs, Mom rests her case: guilty as charged, convicted on grounds of the whole-body lie.

As the daughter grows up, she learns to monitor and mask

many of her own deception cues. She meets her mother's gaze directly, shakes her head sideward, lowers her eyebrows, and keeps her shoulders back to answer, "No—never." Giving fewer bodily signals, her lie is not as visible. But a perceptive mom still notices her daughter's pouted lips, self-clasping hands, pigeon toes, and reddish ears. She detects deceit in what I call a "partial-body lie."

The young woman further hones her skills as an adult. A louder, more convincing "No" rolls off her tongue. Neither flushed ears nor pouted lips belie the word's "truth." Her denial looks more plausible still, yet Mom remains unconvinced.

Could it be her daughter's hands, which are clasped too tightly in her lap, or her iffy pigeon toes? Daughter has no clue that she emits these signals, nor does Mom consciously decode them as signs. Yet both are common deception cues that contrast with the body's natural poise—an unaffected voice, relaxed hands, and toes angled out—while telling the truth. Though she sends fewer deception cues than she did in her teen years, her partial-body lie still confesses: "I'm deceiving you."

Since body movements are harder to edit than words, the tongue makes a better liar. Even the best con man cannot tell a lie without showing some bodily signs of deceit. Surely his mother, at least, could detect something awry. For visible feedback on vocal deception, look to the most informative of all our body parts: the hands, shoulders, lips, and eyes.

A DECEITFUL FLUSH

Becoming red or rosy in the face from embarrassment, shyness, or shame is a deception cue of the sporadic liar. Career liars—underhanded politicians, dishonest CEOs, and those who tell lies for a living—become insensitive, and no longer feel the guilt of liar's remorse.

Facial flushing occurs when one becomes the focus of attention or feels ashamed while deceiving. Suddenly the face, ears, and neck redden. The entire upper chest may turn red in some cases. Those who do not readily blush still show a reddening atop the ears in what I call a "protoblush." A blush or protoblush with a particular line of questioning suggests one may have something to hide.

Blushing is caused by sudden arousal of the sympathetic nervous system, which dilates small blood vessels of the face and body. Some people blush uncontrollably in almost any situation. Their flush, due to shyness or "social phobia," is not usually deceptive. A few suffer such embarrassment that they undergo surgery to interrupt sympathetic-nervous supply to their faces. In a thorascopic sympathectomy, an incision is made through the armpit into the thoracic cavity to sever a nerve located close to the spine's sympathetic chain ganglia. Postoperative faces no longer redden, even while telling lies.

A CASE OF THE FIDGETY DIGITS

On August 17, 1998, President Bill Clinton testified on camera before a federal grand jury about his conduct with White House intern Monica Lewinsky. Reviewing the videotape, it seemed that his hands were on trial rather than Clinton the whole man.

Queries about Clinton's personal life caused his left hand's thumb and four fingers to stiffen and gesture rigidly at the camera. Asked how he would define a sexual relationship, Clinton's hands fiddled nervously with his reading glasses. As his mind groped for answers, his fingers fidgeted in a trivial task at hand.

Bill Clinton looked like a guilty schoolboy in the principal's office. Pausing to think, he clasped his hands and fingers tightly together. He looked anything but presidential as he cradled his chin snugly between supporting, opened palms. The world leader's culpable hands were quite unlike the confident ones we'd grown to know and trust.

Clinton spent a good deal of time holding a water glass, then a soda can, not in an assured "power grip," but limply between the tactile pads of his fingertips in what anthropologists call a "precision grip." If the power grip shows conviction, the precision grip shows a more tentative frame of mind. Finally, after questioning ended, Bill Clinton walked to the Map Room of the White House and admitted that he had, in fact, had an inappropriate sexual relationship with his intern Miss Lewinsky.

> **Hands are such incredibly gifted communicators that they always bear watching, especially in matters of truth or falsehood.**

For those who watched his hands, the president's admission of guilt was hardly news. Hands are the most expressive of all our body parts. They have more to say than faces. Not only do fingers show emotions, depict ideas, and point to butterflies on the wing—they also read Braille, speak in sign languages, and write poetry. Hands are such incredibly gifted communicators that they always bear watching, especially in matters of truth or falsehood.

So connected are hands to the central nervous system that deceivers are unable to keep them still. If there were a first law of nonverbal dynamics it would read, "A hand tends to stay in motion even while at rest." One of the most telling signs of lying takes place when hands engage in what psychologists call "self-stimulating" behaviors, or "self-stim" for short. In these mostly unconscious actions, the digits reach out and touch each other, touch clothing, or handle nearby body parts.

Just as rubbing a sore elbow relieves momentary physical pain, holding one's own hand can relieve psychological pain. Catching a thumb in a drawer, we vigorously rub it to compete with the brain's awareness of our thumb's acute hurt. Caught in a lie, we vigorously self-stim to take our mind off the psychological hurt.

For momentary relief, we unconsciously handle body parts, worry beads, and touch stones when emotions run high. We touch for the sheer psychic comfort and reassurance touching provides. Studies show that self-stimulating behaviors—holding an arm or a wrist, massaging a hand, rubbing or scratching the nose—increase when we feel fearful, doubtful, or deceitful.

Like a polygraph test, self-touching reflects the arousal level of our sympathetic nervous system's fight-or-flight response.

Fidgeting with spectacles, caressing a soda can, or cradling a chin adds sensory input to compete for attention with input from external stressors. If your pointed question bothers me, I seek temporary relief by scratching, rubbing, or kneading a body part. Since the brain's master switching hub, the thalamus, cannot process all incoming signals at once, it selectively admits some while weeding others out. Using the body's paramount touch channel, tactile self-stim reduces anxiety by blocking signals from the visual and auditory channels. Touching the body brings attention inward, away from upsetting sights and sounds outside.

Biologists call self-stimulation a "displacement" behavior. Like human beings, other mammals and birds also displace to relieve the animal equivalent of anxiety. Ducks preen their feathers, cats lick their fur, and chimps scratch their chests when they feel the least bit unnerved.

Primatologist Jane Goodall studied scratching in our nearest animal relatives, the chimpanzees. "The more intense the anxiety or conflict situation," she found, "the more vigorous the scratching becomes. It typically occurred when the chimpanzees are worried or frightened by my presence or that of a high-ranking chimpanzee" (Lawick-Goodall 1968, 329). Goodall's apes strummed their own tactile nerves to relieve what they saw with their eyes.

As in great apes, a human's scratch may not merely satisfy an itch. When scratching starts precisely as one begins to answer a probing question, it's the body's way of saying, "I'm not sure." Fidgety digits that unwittingly coincide with the onset of a verbal denial may signal ambiguity, equivocation, or a kind of double-speak known as the "nondenial denial."

In a nondenial denial, one's spoken words may be "true" without literally denying. Since they are deliberately meant to give a wrong impression, however, they do factually lie. For example, Bill Clinton's statement that he did not have sexual relations with Monica Lewinsky was a nondenial denial, because his personal definition of sex precluded the oral variety.

The phrase "nondenial denial" was coined in the Watergate era by Bob Woodward and Carl Bernstein in their book *All the President's Men* as a label for evasive statements made by then U.S. attorney general John Mitchell. At televised Watergate hearings in 1973, Mitchell repeatedly touched his mouth and eyes while denying involvement in the Watergate burglary. This led some TV viewers at the time, including body-language expert and psychotherapist R. Don Steele, to detect deception in Mitchell's remarks. Steele may have been right, because on January 1, 1975, Mitchell, America's former top cop, was convicted on federal charges of conspiracy, perjury, and obstruction of justice. He served nineteen months in prison.

DECODING A LIP TOUCH

Worldwide, the most frequent self-stim behavior may be the lip touch, a brief or sustained stimulation of the highly sensitive fleshy folds around the mouth. The lip touch is delivered to one or both lips with the knuckles, fingers, or fingertips, or with an object such as a pencil or pen held in the hand. If you see a lip touch in someone who answers a probing question, take note. You may be witness to a lie in progress.

CASE OF THE LIFTED SHOULDERS

On October 5, 2000, truck driver William Bradley "Brad" Jackson of Spokane, Washington, was convicted of first-degree murder for the death of his nine-year-old daughter, Valiree. Upon his conviction, Jackson, thirty-four, showed no emotion.

A year earlier, on October 18, 1999, a crying and shaking Brad Jackson ran from house to house in his neighborhood, seemingly panic-stricken that Valiree was missing. Suspecting foul play, Spokane police officers attached global-positioning devices to Jackson's vehicles. Brad then unknowingly led officers, via satellite imagery, to where Valiree's body was buried in a shallow grave.

At his murder trial, Jackson was convicted of suffocating Valiree with a bed pillow. Earlier, he testified that she had died from an overdose of the antidepressant drug Paxil. Jackson told jurors that since nobody would have believed he was innocent, he buried his daughter's body, then returned to his neighborhood and reported her missing.

Deputy prosecutor Jack Driscoll stated that exposing Brad Jackson's string of lies was what ultimately led to a conviction in the case. "His credibility was a factor for us," Driscoll said. As I watched local TV coverage of Brad Jackson's trial, the credibility factor that stood out most to me was the man's elevated shoulders. Jackson's shoulders visibly shrugged with each and every answer. His shoulder shrugs were frequent and, by any nonverbal standard, exaggerated. For an adult, they were the most amplified shrugs I'd ever seen. Jackson's shoulders repeatedly rose and fell like ocean waves crashing upon the sands of his credibility. His words said one thing; his shoulders said another.

Shoulders are the paired, jointed organs that connect the arms to the torso. The flexibility and visibility of human shoulders, and the fact that the upper trapezius muscle that moves them is linked—like our throat's voice box—to emotionally sensitive special visceral nerves, make them highly expressive as signs of uncertainty and deception. The upper trapezius is governed by the accessory nerve (cranial XI), a special visceral nerve that also controls the larynx. While a person is answering questions on the witness stand, shoulder shrugs, throat clearing, and vocal tension can reveal deception all at the same time.

Anatomically, the bones of our shoulder girdle consist of two flattened shoulder blades (or scapulas), each connected to a bracing collarbone (or clavicle). The sides of the bony girdle sit on our rib cage like shoulder pads. Unattached to any bones but the clavicles, the scapulas glide up and down, move back and forth, and rotate about our back and spine. Since only the clavicles' attachments to the breastbone stabilize their motion, they are highly mobile. And like Pinocchio's growing nose, shoulders grow higher when we tell a lie.

The shoulder shrug is a universal sign of psychological uncertainty. Shrug cues modify, counteract, or contradict verbal remarks. With the statement "Yes, I'm sure," a lifted shoulder suggests, "I'm not so sure." A shrug reveals misleading, ambiguous, or uncertain areas in dialogue and oral testimony, and thus provides a visual opportunity to probe for misstatements, exaggerations, and lies. Though Brad Jackson ultimately apologized for lying in court, he still claimed that he did not kill his daughter. His shoulders, it appears, claimed otherwise.

UNCERTAIN HAND SHRUGS

On May 7, 2006, I turned on the TV to watch a Seattle Mariners baseball game. By chance, the channel was tuned to MSNBC's *Headliners and Legends*, which was showing old footage of a handsome young man making a statement to police about a murder in New York's Central Park. However, something about the man's explanation seemed self-serving, both disingenuous and misleading. As I watched more carefully, I traced the seeming lack of candor to his hands.

As the man explained it, the victim, an eighteen-year-old woman he'd just met in a bar, had (1) been the aggressor in their sex play at the park, (2) tied up his arms with her panties, and (3) died accidentally when he flipped her over his shoulder. He accented each of his speaking points with hand shrugs.

A hand shrug is a palm-up gesture that originates from the larger shoulder-shrug display. In the hand shrug, the hand is fully open, the fingers extended, and the palm lifted upward to an appealing, imploring, or "begging" position.

It turned out that the young man was Robert E. Chambers—known in the 1980s as the "Preppy Killer." Chambers pled guilty to first-degree manslaughter for the August 26, 1986, strangulation death of Jennifer Levin, and was sentenced to fifteen years in prison in April 1988.

That he'd seemed less than convincing in his videotaped police interview was due to the frequent hand shrugs of uncertainty that graphically belied the certitude of his words. By "begging" police to believe him, he telegraphed that his alibi could not stand up on merit alone. If he wasn't confident in his own words, why should the police be? Robert Chambers's hands quite literally begged the question of truth.

READING LIPS

Lips are brutally honest. When we lie, our lips visibly tighten, roll in, and compress. Despite one's best effort to control it, a compressed-lips facial expression is utterly frank. To illustrate the innate ability of lips to belie a lie, witness another Bill Clinton example. His body language through the Monica Lewinsky years was so well documented and observed by so many millions on TV that his deceitful demeanor has become a textbook case of what nonverbal deception looks like.

In June 1995, Monica Lewinsky, twenty-one, came to the White House in Washington, D.C., to serve as an unpaid intern. On January 21, 1998, national news media reported an alleged sexual relationship between Lewinsky and President Clinton. The president publicly denied the affair. On January 23, 1998, Clinton reassured his cabinet that he'd not had an affair. Three days later came the famous televised denial, in which he pointed his index finger at the American people.

Throughout the Lewinsky scandal, I watched President Clinton's lips. They told a most revealing tale. His lips visibly pressed together, tightened, and rolled into a thin line each time he talked with reporters about the Lewinsky affair. Clinton's tight-lipped facial expression jumped out at me. When several members of his cabinet compressed their lips on camera, too, while upholding the president's innocence, I knew it must be true: our president was lying.

Then came the graphic AP photos of President Clinton sitting in the Map Room of the White House on August 17, 1998, minutes before making his apology to the world. A major presidential lip clench, with obvious tension showing around the mouth, was captured moments before he shamefully admitted, "Indeed, I did have a relationship with Miss Lewinsky that was not appropriate."

If hands are our most expressive bodily features, lips are our most emotional. The latter compress, tighten, and press together through contraction of the lips' orbicularis oris muscles and the lower jaw's masseter. Lip and jaw tension clearly reflects anxious feelings, nervousness, and emotional stress. In the context of Clinton's emotion-charged admission to the secret affair, compressed lips clearly signaled his guilt. Perhaps it was not the lie that caused his lips to tighten, but the shame of being caught.

GUILTY LIPS

Compressed lips are a gestural fossil left over from early mammalian evolution. The tense-mouth display is governed by special visceral nerves originally designed for feeding. Lip compression is emotionally responsive today and reflects visceral sensations— "gut feelings"—aroused by powerful sentiments of anger, remorse, shame, or guilt. In effect, we tighten our lips protectively to seal off the mouth opening from real or imagined harm. Emotional stimuli pass from higher brain centers to centers below, where the facial nerve (cranial VII) arises in the brain stem. From deep within the brain stem, the facial nerve travels out of the skull and links to the mouth's orbicularis oris muscles, which tighten, compress, and roll in our lips for all to see.

EVASIVE EYES

On August 2, 2002, Boston cardinal Bernard F. Law testified in Suffolk Superior Court on matters of a settlement agreement with alleged victims of sexual abuse by priests. According to *Boston Globe* reporter Kathleen Burge, Law appeared to be comfortable on the witness stand, yet between questions "he looked down at his clasped hands" (Burge 2002).

Recall Bill Clinton's clasped hands, one of several self-stimulating behaviors he used while testifying about his conduct with Monica Lewinsky. In isolation, clasped hands do not a liar make. But when a witness simultaneously clasps and looks down— avoids eye contact by gazing downward—suspicion is raised.

Shortly after New Year's Day in 2002, some eight months before gazing down at his own clasped hands, Cardinal Law telephoned one of his most trusted advisers, businessman Jack Connors Jr. Law asked for Connors's advice just before national news about the Boston archdiocese's first major sex scandal involving priests was to break. Connors advised Law, in no uncertain terms, to tell the whole truth. But when Connors asked the cardinal if he knew about any other child-abusing priests, Law answered only that "there might be one or two" (Ferdinand and Duggan 2002).

In 2003, Law's Boston archdiocese reached an $85 million settlement agreement with more than five hundred priest-abuse victims. Though Cardinal Law was never charged with a crime, Massachusetts attorney general Thomas Reilly officially concluded in a ninety-one-page report chronicling the investigation into how church leaders handled the scandal that Law bore "ultimate responsibility for the tragic treatment of children that occurred during his tenure." The cardinal's downturned eyes on the witness stand a year earlier may have reflected chagrin about his role in the scandal.

In matters of truth and falsehood, we finely attune to the direction of eyes. Contrast between colored irises and the prominent whites of our eyes, anthropologists maintain, enables us to gauge accurately where others are looking. In two worldwide studies carried out in seventy-five countries and forty-three languages, researchers found that most people think liars avert their gaze while deceiving (Global Deception Research Team 2006). With intimations of embarrassment, shame, and guilt, downward eye aversion on the witness stand can be a telling sign of deceit.

> **What ails you that you keep gazing on the ground?**
> —Dante, *Purgatorio,* canto 19

We may bow our heads to gaze down or rotate our eyeballs downward in their sockets. Gazing down may convey a defeated attitude and reflect guilt, shame, or submissiveness while distorting the truth or telling a lie. Gazing down while saying "I am innocent" shows a speaker may not believe his own words. True statements are likely to be given with a confident, face-to-face, level gaze.

In some cultures a downward gaze does not automatically indicate a lie. In Japan, people are taught to focus on a speaker's neck in order to avoid eye contact. In Mexico, young men learn to drop their eyes when Father scolds, lest they seem disrespectful. Nonetheless, when a handcuffed suspect gazes down, bows his head, and covers his face and eyes under a shirt as police lead him away, a reasonable deduction from body language points to guilt.

On April 5, 2006, the Associated Press reported that "Doyle was bent over in the front seat of the police vehicle in an apparent attempt to hide his face" (Spitzer 2006). The suspect in question was Brian J. Doyle, fifty-five, who was arrested the day before at his Silver Spring, Maryland, home on charges of using a computer to seduce someone he believed to be a fourteen-year-old girl. Since Doyle was the deputy press secretary for the U.S. Department of Homeland Security at the time, the guilt, remorse, and possible embarrassment revealed by his lowered head may have been markedly greater than had he been just an ordinary John Doe.

On CNN footage of the April 4 arrest, I watched Mr. Doyle bow his head and face fully away to his left, to avoid news cameras, as police led him away in cuffs. Seeing the head bow, I detected a powerful sense of shame. In news photos taken at his Florida trial, I saw a magnified head bow, bent forward at a forty-five-degree angle above his clasped hands on the defense table, as his lawyer comforted him in court. The man's spectacular fall from grace was reflected in the crestfallen head posture. On November 17, 2006, former Homeland Security official Brian Doyle was sentenced to five years in a Florida prison, to be followed by ten years' probation and the obligation to register as a sex offender.

Bowing the head forward is assisted by the backbone's erector spinae muscles, which are supplied directly by spinal nerves rather than by more evolved nerve plexuses that are subject to deliberate control. The bow's submissive tone stems from the role these muscles and nerves originally played in curling the head and trunk forward into a protective crouch. Head lowering and back rounding in response to an arrest connote "spineless" surrender and acceptance of blame.

You will notice that head bowing is accompanied by downcast eyes. The six muscles that cooperate to move each eyeball are common to all vertebrates. Direct eye contact (or "primary gaze," i.e., looking straight ahead) involves all six muscles. Gazing down occurs as the inferior rectus muscle, which is governed by the oculomotor nerve (cranial III), contracts as the prime mover. Shameful or guilty feelings move our eyes downward through protective circuits established millions of years ago in lower, sub-cortical vision centers of the human midbrain. Voluntarily gazing down involves higher brain centers of the prefrontal eye fields.

According to Whitewater special prosecutor Kenneth Starr, "There is no substitute for looking a witness in the eye." Starr is right, but since many criminals also know that gaze aversion is a deception cue, they may manage to maintain eye contact on pur-pose. To seem truthful, pedophiles will prolong eye contact with a victim's parents. As CIA operative David Forden advised Poland's Colonel Ryszard Kuklinski, a secret informant, "If someone should surprise you, stay calm. Look him right in the eye—always maintain eye contact. That way you don't look shifty-eyed, but, more important, all he will notice is your eyes" (Chelminski 1999). Lying eyes may not always be what they seem.

CAUGHT IN A DOOZY

In 1922, T. S. Eliot wrote, "April is the cruelest month." April 2003 marked the publication of James Frey's purportedly nonfic-tion book, *A Million Little Pieces* (New York: Doubleday). The book is an autobiographical memoir about an angry young man's survival against desperate odds in the world of alcoholism, drug addiction, and crime. A self-described tough guy, Frey purport-edly had root canals without Novocain, fought with police, spent months in jail, and ultimately found his girlfriend dead by her own hand, a suicide by hanging.

In October 2005, TV talk-show host Oprah Winfrey publicly endorsed *A Million Little Pieces* and picked it for her book club. Winfrey's endorsement boosted Frey's book sales into the millions.

On January 8, 2006, the Smoking Gun Web site posted as its lead article "The Man Who Conned Oprah." According to the article, "Police reports, court records, interviews with law enforcement personnel, and other sources have put the lie to many key sections of Frey's book."

On January 26, 2006, James Frey, thirty-six, appeared as a guest on *The Oprah Winfrey Show*. With her left hand tightly balled into a fist, Oprah accused Frey of telling multiple lies in his book. He did not spend months in jail, as he'd written, but just a few hours in a police station. His girlfriend did not hang herself, as he'd professed. He did not have two root canals without Novocain, as he'd claimed.

Frey answered Oprah's question about his extreme dental work—which he'd used to show he was tough enough to withstand severe pain—with the statement that, in writing the book, he had "struggled with the idea of it."

"No, the lie of it," Oprah shot back. "That's a lie. It's not an idea, James, that's a lie." Frey meekly confessed, "Yes." If Frey's physical pain in the dental chair was fantasy, his emotional pain while sitting on Oprah's couch was real. His head bowed forward, his eyebrows lifted, his eyes widened, his eyeballs rolled downward, his mouth tightened and his lips compressed, his shoulders slumped forward, and his hands clasped in his lap with fingers tightly intertwined. Whether he felt guilt, embarrassment, or both, he gave off many signals of the whole-body lie.

Judging from his body language, Frey's sympathetic nervous system was in full-scale flight mode. His laryngeal voice box tensed. His mouth became dry. He repeatedly sipped from a water glass held in his left hand, with fingers in the tentative precision grip. Vocal pauses were filled with ums and ahs. His sitting posture—left ankle crossed over right knee—was fixed and immobile, frozen in place. He gave very few hand gestures as he spoke, and did not nod to affirm key speaking points.

Viewers including me watched author Frey twist in the web of his admitted lies. He was accused of conning Oprah Winfrey, one of television's most famous personalities. Frey's body language clearly revealed to millions the truth of his deceit.

We have seen that hands, shoulders, lips, and eyes can give off surefire signals that someone is lying. Here are some key cues that can point to deception:

- Sudden reddening about the face, ears, and neck
- Onset of the fidgety digits
- Self-stimulation with fingers and hands
- Chronic shoulder and palm shrugs
- Compressed, tightened, in-rolled lips
- Gaze aversion downward
- Vocal pauses filled with ums and ahs

In the next chapter, we will decipher the body language of some of the best criminal deceivers, con men, including that of the notorious "Dr. John" from Ghana, "the richest man in the world."

3

MARKS OF THE SWINDLER

O what a goodly outside falsehood hath!

—SHAKESPEARE, *The Merchant of Venice*

SWINDLING IS ABOUT theatrics, props, and sleight of hand. When the stage is properly set, the intended victim or "mark" enters, and money changes hands. Verbally, con men are smooth, persuasive, and articulate, but 99 percent of their charm is nonverbal. A swindler's poise is in body language, facial expressions, and posturing.

The earliest con men date back to the early urban centers of ancient Egypt and Mesopotamia. In anonymous city settings, imposters could gain the confidence of well-to-do strangers, prey on their greed to get something for nothing, and leave town before the bamboozled marks could get even. A typical swindle was perpetrated in games of chance, such as dice. Found in northern Iraq, the earliest known six-sided die, made of baked clay marked with numerical dots or "pips," dates back to 2750 BC. Soon after, throughout the Middle East, dishonest gamblers began using loaded dice to beat the odds. As their scams came to light, the itinerant con men simply packed up their dice and moved on.

Another ancient gambling scam, the thimblerig or shell game, dates back to at least the Middle Ages. Played with a tiny ball or pellet and three small nutshells, cups, or thimbles, the illegal game is easily hidden in one's pocket should police come calling. Players gamble on which of the three nutshells covers the pellet, after the game's owner has thoroughly shuffled and moved the shells around.

Shell-game owners use clever prestidigitation, or "quick finger" movements, to maneuver a pellet from shell to shell faster than the eye can see. Thus, most marks are bound to lose their bets. Should a savvy mark catch on to the trick, planted accomplices in the crowd push forward and shoulder him out of the game.

The principle of hiding pellets, peas, or soft little balls in primitive shell games has been likened to hiding huge amounts of cash in modern accounting schemes. WorldCom and Enron come to mind. Underlying all shell games, big or small, is the maxim that the hand moves quicker than the eye.

More correctly, the hand moves quicker than the cerebral cortex. The shell gamer's nimble digits make incredibly precise movements on a stage blooming with visual confusion. There is far too much for two eyes to see, and the pea gets lost in the shuffle. As we will see below, the neurology of sight is vastly more complex than the neurology of hand movements.

Light reflected from the pellet, the nutshells, and the con artist's hands cast tiny images on the eye's nerve-sensitive retina. From here, electrochemical impulses cable through the optic nerve to a visual area at the very back of the brain. Neurons in this region respond to linear details and to wavelengths of color. A second visual area enhances our image of the game's linear and color details. Additional processing takes place for the recognition of form, movement, and extra details of color. Diverse areas of the brain's cerebral cortex then must cooperate to unify and give meaning to our overall vision of the game. In short, so much mental processing goes on while watching the shell game that certain details are left sight unseen. Just where the little ball hides is anybody's guess.

Meanwhile, the practiced, seemingly invisible hand movements that move the ball from shell to shell are controlled, not by the cerebral cortex, but by more ancient motor centers acquired millions of years earlier. Called the basal ganglia, these brain areas are less complicated than the cortex but are still very fast, very efficient, and virtually automatic. Once the game's operator learns to shuffle the nutshells, his basal ganglia take control. With practice, shuffling becomes as easy and automatic as brushing one's teeth.

The shell game's owner has a distinct neurological advantage. It's simply easier for his brain to move the pea than for yours to track its movement.

BODY LANGUAGE OF CARNIVAL CON ARTISTS

To decipher the body language of modern-day swindlers, we begin with the colorful clothing, gaudy demeanor, and beckoning gestures of the carnival con artist. Every nonverbal basic of swindling is here, from the showy first meeting to the conspiratorial wink to the final pocketing of cash. Carnival "agents," as they refer to themselves, attract attention with blinking lights, flashy show-business clothes, and noisy calling: "Come on over, break a balloon, win a prize!" Vocal calls are animated with lively gestures of the hands. Among them, writes Peter Fenton, author of *Eyeing the Flash*, are "the bread-and-butter beckoning wave of the full hand; the classy wave with all fingers closed except for the pinkie, which [is] fluttered; and the pissed-off bird with all fingers closed but for the middle" (Fenton 2005, 125).

Agents recognize the natural persuasiveness of hand gestures. Attention-getting hand movements compete with the buzzing, blooming confusion of the midway. Showing an open palm is a universal way to say, "I mean no harm." Reaching out a friendly opened hand establishes a personal link that draws people spatially and emotionally closer. Since nerve cells in the brain's temporal lobes are innately programmed to notice finger positions and hand shapes, we respond to gestures with great alertness. Marks instinctively take note of a carnie's beckoning hands.

Like a welcoming palm, the midway's entrance is also designed to look friendly. Harmless balloon-dart, duck-pond, and goldfish-toss games for children invite you to enter a child-friendly space. In such a setting, who could possibly cheat you? The answer, of course, is anyone and everyone. Flashy prizes beckon, but "prizes" are worth less than what you pay to play the game. In the duck-pond bet, for example, each floating bird has a number inscribed on its underside. Most numbers will earn you a cheap plastic toy, ring, or whistle. The duck with the trophy-prize-winning number—for the color TV—may be hidden in a tunnel, out of play, until the agent's hand releases it with a secret lever.

Should a crowd of angry marks gather to question the duck pond's integrity—and threaten to call police—a supervisor comes forward to calm the mob down. Should his words and gestures fail, he calls on a confederate, an actor known as a "shill," who offers to buy as many chances to win the color TV as there are ducks in the pond. Money changes hands, the hidden duck is released, and the shill "wins." The big prize is triumphantly carried away atop his shoulders as the duped crowd cheers. All is well again at the duck pond.

Thirty minutes later, the confederate returns the TV for a full refund. The flashy prop has played its role in the con game one more time. As in the shell game, unruly marks have been "shouldered aside."

At carnivals, as in more sophisticated confidence-game venues, the main goal is establishing trust. On the midway, carnies broker trust with each other nonverbally through touching. A former teenage carnival con man, Peter Fenton describes how an older con man named "Horserace" put his arm around the teen's neck to wheedle a loan: "Could you front me for a double sawbuck? Pay you back the exact minute we count up tonight" (Fenton 2005, 121). Knowing how often carnies con carnies, Peter passed on his fellow agent's touch. No money changed hands.

TOUCH AND FEELING

Touch cues are powerfully real. If seeing is believing, touching is knowing for sure. A tap, ding, or "soft touch" on the forearm when asking to borrow money transcends a purely verbal request. The touch adds feeling to make the matter more personal. Touch cues are used worldwide to show emotion in child care, and later in adulthood to establish rapport in courtship. A gentle hand laid on a shoulder shows fondness. A carnie's touch shows fondness for your wallet.

BODY LANGUAGE OF THE WORLD'S ULTIMATE CON MAN

Let's move from shell games and carnivals to big-time scams, where the take is measured in millions rather than tens of dollars.

Though the stakes are significantly higher, we will see that body language is significantly the same.

Dr. John Ackah Blay-Miezah, originally of Ghana, called himself the richest man in the world, with a secret trust fund of $27 billion. Nonverbally, in clothing (Savile Row suit, Charvet shirt, gold cuff links), architecture (iron-gated home in London, spacious office in Piccadilly), and vehicle (ivory Rolls-Royce), Dr. John had the look and feel of a very wealthy man.

In words, he variously declared himself to be the son, nephew, or cousin of Ghana's deposed president Kwame Nkrumah. Nkrumah had set up the trust fund and supposedly named Blay-Miezah as its sole beneficiary.

In deeds, Blay-Miezah sat on a tribal throne, cloaked his body in ceremonial robes, and performed a solemn African ritual in which he vowed to speak only the truth.

The ritual was witnessed, in person, by the late Ed Bradley of CBS's *60 Minutes*. Blay-Miezah daubed Beefeater gin on his throne and spat the liquor three times on his staff. In tandem with the flamboyant messages given off by Blay-Miezah's clothing, regal architecture, and ivory Rolls-Royce, his ritualistic body movements targeted gullible aspects of the right brain hemisphere, which is far more emotional and willing to believe than is the coolly rational, guarded, more skeptical left.

By ceremonially spitting three times on his staff, Blay-Miezah ritually invoked a biological principle called "rhythmic repetition." The rote repetition ensured that his message would be received. In communications theory this is known as "redundancy." The rhythmic quality of his repetition added feeling. It evoked an emotional atmosphere in which participants would share a ritualistic, lower level of cognitive functioning. Overall, the rite's rhythmic theatrics induced a momentary, mesmerizing suspension of disbelief.

HIDDEN MEANING IN REPEATED MOVEMENT

Highly stylized, rhythmic repetition—a ballerina's pirouette, a priest's formalized sprinkling of holy water, a sumo wrestler's ceremonial stomp in the ring—captures attention, extends the nonverbal signal in time, and makes any message seem more important. Rhythmic repetition is an important rapport-building signal in courtship. Lizards bob heads in tandem to court, dogs wag tails in synchrony, and humans dance together to join as pairs.

Repeated movement stimulates an emotional response that can be mesmerizing. The rhythmic wigwag of windshield wipers, the flicker of candlelight, and the singsong melody of an arcane incantation can induce a trancelike, hypnotic state. In fact, the nonverbal key to hypnosis lies in the rhythmic repetition of body movements, gestures, and sounds that match the natural pattern of brain waves.

Rhythmic repetition is key to the con man's world as well. Nutshells shuffle back and forth, carnies repeat droning calls, African "heirs" perform fanciful rituals. The hidden aim of reiteration is to draw marks subliminally into the con.

When Dr. John promised to return investors not less than 1,000 percent on their investments in the scheme to "unlock" his trust fund, many believed. It is estimated that he attracted $250 million from gullible investors around the world. Yet, though many waited for years, none received a dime. Dr. John's nonverbal magic was strong. He looked investors right in the eye and promised to pay. Invoking rhythmic repetition in words, he vowed "never, never, never, never" to dishonor his promise.

Dr. John Ackah Blay-Miezah of Ghana died in June of 1992. His was an extreme case of swindling, but the nonverbal basics of his charm typify every successful scam. Swindlers package their words in mesmerizing, smoke-and-mirror facades of posture, prop, and dramatic posing. There is a flurry of hand gestures, a momentary suspension of disbelief, and money changes hands.

Their nonverbal pretenses make swindlers the most entertaining of all criminals.

CHARMED, I'M SURE

As well as being very good actors, confidence men are very gifted charmers. They beguile, entrance, and captivate you to take your money. Many con men are also irresistible and prey as bigamists upon women they seek to marry for profit. A great deal of a bigamist-swindler's sex appeal comes from clothing and adornment. The actor carefully sets his stage and enters, in full costume, dressed as a knight in shining armor. But when a fake knight vies for his maiden's hand in marriage too soon, shortly after the first meeting, alarm bells should sound.

In the case of counterfeit Navy SEAL Eric Cooper, the costume was a crisp white naval uniform. The symbolic meanings of white—solemnity, purity, and fidelity—became him. Cooper's victims, many of whom married the pretend naval officer, found his charm and uniform irresistible (Dahler 2005). Over a ten-year period, serial spouse Cooper married or became engaged to nine different women within just weeks of meeting them for the very first time (Anonymous 2006b).

On August 8, 2006, Eric Eugene Cooper, thirty, was found guilty of illegally altering wife Krystal Weber's vehicle title, and was sentenced in a Harris County, Texas, court to fifteen years in prison (Parsons 2006). Several of Cooper's wives and girlfriends testified at his trial, where a picture emerged of a deceptive con man who masqueraded as a Navy officer and heir to a multimillion-dollar trust fund.

Ex-wife Krystal, twenty-four, told how she'd met Eric on a singles Web site. After a whirlwind courtship in which Eric claimed to be a U.S. Naval Academy graduate, a Navy jet pilot, and a former Navy SEAL, they married in Las Vegas (O'Hare 2006). Other women told of his Navy theme. An ex-girlfriend said she'd seen Eric carrying a military M16 rifle, and a third woman said she saw Eric in a white uniform speaking to an elementary school class (O'Hare 2006).

Cooper played a convincing charmer in his character role as a naval officer. The flaw in his performance was that instead of a cast of dozens, there was a cast of only one. His was a solo performance, and the pseudo SEAL's white uniform stood out, by itself, as an anomaly. That there were no shipmates whatsoever should have raised suspicions. Indeed, the stand-alone uniform, hasty marriage proposals, and trick trust fund were loud and clear crime signals in Cooper's plot to win money by matrimony.

CON WITH THE COOLEST DEMEANOR

Lying is the confidence man's bread and butter. Little wonder, then, that con men are among the best deceivers in the world of crime. One of the twentieth century's very best liars was the American writer Clifford Irving, who authored a fraudulent book—*The Autobiography of Howard Hughes*—and sold it to McGraw-Hill, one of America's most distinguished publishing houses, for $750,000.

In face-to-face meetings, Clifford Irving lied to—and successfully fooled—McGraw-Hill, *Life* magazine, and veteran TV interviewer Mike Wallace of CBS's *60 Minutes*. Irving claimed to have exclusive rights to the reclusive billionaire's life story, which, Irving further lied, Hughes had asked him to write.

So believable were Irving's words and demeanor that on December 7, 1971, McGraw-Hill bought the rights to his book. But when the publisher announced the book's debut, Howard Hughes came out of seclusion and lodged a very vocal protest. On January 7, 1972, Hughes talked by telephone from his Bahamas retreat to a press conference held in North Hollywood, California. Hughes, who did not appear on camera, said, "I don't know him [Irving]. I never saw him. I never even heard of him until days ago when this came to my attention" (Brown and Broeske 1996, 351). In response, Irving claimed the disembodied voice heard on TV was not really Hughes's. McGraw-Hill, too, claimed the press conference was a fraud.

On January 16, 1972, Irving sat for an interview with Mike Wallace on *60 Minutes*. Though he remained cool and looked perfectly believable, Irving lied (convincingly, according to Wallace) about every detail of the bogus Hughes "autobiography." Soon after, Clifford Irving's con completely collapsed and the chastened novelist confessed. Subsequently, on June 16, 1972, Clifford and wife Edith, his partner in crime, were found guilty in U.S. federal court on numerous criminal counts, including perjury, forgery, and fraud. *Time* magazine named Irving "Con Man of the Year." After serving seventeen months in prison, Irving was released in February 1974.

Twenty-five years later, on May 19, 1999, Clifford Irving sat for a second interview with Mike Wallace on a CBS special, *60 Minutes Classics: The Con Men*. Revisiting the first *60 Minutes* tape, Wallace noted that Irving looked "extremely relaxed and confident" (Jackman 2003, 52). Irving himself confessed he could feel his heart "fluttering" at the initial meeting, and that he'd "clutched his manuscript against his chest for protection" (Jackman 2003, 52).

In the second TV interview, Clifford Irving revealed the secret of his lying success. He'd remained so cool because he believed he was telling the truth: "You wondered how I could lie so fluently to you," Irving told Wallace. "That's because at some level, I believed everything I was telling you. I believed we [Howard Hughes and I] met" (Jackman 2003, 54).

STILL LIFE WITH CHARM

Con artists prey in a very vocal, very visual world. Voice tones are intimate, dominant, insistent, and charming. The con man courts you like a trusted friend or lover. Body movements are smooth, practiced, ceremonial, and dramatic. Nutshells shuffle, hands beckon, ancient rituals repeat. The confidence game slowly entrances you.

One of the most charming con men of recent times was the Hungarian art forger Elmyr de Hory. A flamboyant gentleman, European "nobleman," and rogue boulevardier, de Hory was known for his stylish clothing, gold monocle, and unmatched ability to produce quick forgeries of artwork by the likes of Braque, Magritte, and Picasso. In his 1969 book, *Fake*, author Clifford Irving—who presumably told the truth before his Howard Hughes caper—described de Hory, a fellow resident on the Spanish island of Ibiza, as lovable and "charming" (Jackman 2003, 57). Though often a good thing, in con games charm has a downside. As Gavin de Becker, one of the world's leading experts in predicting criminal behavior, points out: "Charm is almost always a directed instrument, which, like rapport building, has motive. To charm is to compel, to control by allure or attraction" (de Becker 1997, 56).

De Becker, author of *The Gift of Fear: Survival Signals*, rightly likens charm to rapport. Rapport is a pleasant feeling of mutual trust, affinity, and friendship established through verbal and nonverbal means. Nonverbally, rapport shows in shared body movements and postures, in mutually aligned upper bodies, in mutual eye contact, in opened-palm speaking gestures, and in affirmative eyebrow flashes, head nods of agreement, shared laughter, simultaneous shoulder shrugs, and reciprocal smiles. Around the world, these are the cues we send and receive in courtship to woo our mates, or in business to solicit clients.

Elmyr de Hory used his native Hungarian charm to build rapport with the marks who would buy his forgeries. He flew from Paris to New York, Los Angeles, and Brazil selling his fake paintings and drawings. He talked smoothly to strangers at curbside cafés, and threw parties wherever he went.

"The subtlety of making impressions," businessman Mark Mc-Cormack wrote, "demands self-awareness" (McCormack 1984, 27). De Hory's first conniving impression was made in Paris in April 1946, when a wealthy acquaintance, Lady Campbell, visited his home and spotted a line drawing of a girl's head. "Isn't that a Picasso?" she asked. Crime writer Brian Innes describes Elmyr's solicitous reply: "He just sighed tragically and agreed reluctantly to sell it. Lady Campbell was hardly out the door before he had dashed off seven similar drawings" (Innes 2005, 79).

A sigh is a long, deep, audible exhalation given in weariness, sadness, or grief. In 1958, linguists began studying the sigh as an emotional vocalization. To sigh, they learned, is human. The audible, nonverbal sigh is a universal form of "paralanguage"— vocalizations without the grammar of language. Studies of paralanguage have found that vocal pauses, hems, haws, gasps, coughs, throat clearings, and sighs carry meaningful information about unsaid, veiled, or hidden feelings. De Hory's tragic sigh was a typical con man's ploy to fake an emotion for ill-gotten gain.

The elegant body language of Elmyr de Hory's drawings also suggested feeling. In June 1955, Agnes Mongan of Harvard University's Fogg Art Museum bought a drawing she thought was the work of Henri Matisse. Unfortunately, *A Lady with Flowers and Pomegranates* was drawn in 1944 by none other than Elmyr de Hory (Reed 2004). De Hory the charmer had never met Agnes the buyer face-to-face. The splendidly drawn body language of the figure's direct gaze, tilted head, and pensive left hand touching her cheek spoke for itself.

De Hory's artful deceptions ended in December 1976. Facing extradition for fraud from Ibiza, his isle of retreat, Elmyr died at home from an overdose of sleeping pills (Innes 2005, 84). His success as an art forger was due partly to the eloquence of his own body language, and partly to the acknowledged eloquence of his artwork. When you really like somebody—or something—you can easily be fooled by theatrics, props, and sleight of hand.

The body language and demeanor of swindlers is entertaining and generally safe. Their practiced routines are designed to take your money, not your life. To keep your money safe from skillful, shifty scoundrels who may be swindling you, watch for the following crime signals:

- Strangers who smile, touch, and seem too friendly too soon
- Overly dramatic, ceremonial mannerisms and flamboyant body language
- Rehearsed or theatrical hand gestures

· Showy clothing, pretentious physical props
· Conspicuous charm, unusually cool demeanor
· Rhythmic, repetitious rituals

Like snake charmers, con men use repetition to beguile victims before taking their money. In chapter 4, you will learn about the body language of snakes themselves—those who take human lives.

4

A SILENT CRY: THE KILLER'S WARNING SIGNS

And Scott is there, and he's not quite himself again.

—ANNE BIRD, describing Laci Peterson's baby
shower on December 10, 2002

ON JULY 31, 1966, friends noted a change in Charles Whitman. A generally troubled man, he had become "unusually quiet" and seemed uncharacteristically "calm and in good spirits." According to his biographer Gary Lavergne, earlier that day Charles had conclusively resolved to become a mass murderer.

As a boy, Whitman was fascinated by guns and knives. "As soon as he could hold [a gun]," Lavergne wrote, "he did. One infamous photograph shows Charlie as a toddler holding two rifles—one a bolt action, the other a pump." Whitman displayed a pattern of what I call "weapons fancy," the desire to touch, pick up, handle, own, collect, display, and use armaments of efficient design. In patients with frontal-lobe lesions, the mere sight of a knife or firearm is, according to neurologist Marsel Mesulam, "likely to elicit the automatic compulsion to use it" (Mesulam

1992, 697). Neuroscientist Rhawn Joseph has conjectured that Whitman may have had such lesions.

As a teen, Whitman lived in a well-to-do but troubled household in Lake Worth, Florida. His ill-tempered father disciplined him with belts, paddles, and fists. In June 1959, Charles's father beat him for drunkenness, nearly drowning the teenager in the backyard pool (MacLeod 2005). Soon after, Charlie joined the Marines and left home for boot camp. In the Marine Corps, he received training in marksmanship and earned a sharpshooter's badge. He stood out for his ability to hit moving targets.

On September 15, 1961, Whitman became a student at the University of Texas in Austin on a Marine Corps scholarship. He married on August 17, 1962, and began physically abusing his wife, Kathy, as his father had abused his own spouse, Margaret, before. In February of the following year, poor grades coupled with less-than-perfect behavior (angrily threatening to "kick the teeth out" of a fellow soldier) prompted the Marines to withdraw his scholarship. Seven months later, he was court-martialed on charges of gambling and usury, and sentenced to thirty days in the brig. Finally, after an honorable discharge on December 4, 1964, Charlie returned to Austin and college.

When Kathy Whitman noticed Charlie's increasingly depressed mental state, she suggested that he seek counseling. On March 29, 1966, one doctor prescribed Valium. Charlie told another doctor about his recurring homicidal fantasy, one that involved climbing the University of Texas Tower. However, he'd been telling this story for years, and no one, including the doctor, took him seriously.

Sometime before or after his psychiatric counseling, Charlie took a giant misstep backward and began using the potent amphetamine Dexedrine. Then, on July 22, 1966, Whitman visited the tower observation deck with his brother, John. The crime signals were piling up.

On July 31, 1966, the increasingly agitated Charles Whitman suddenly reached a point of calm, as his friends noticed just hours before the crime. *"From that moment on,"* Lavergne wrote, *"he became extraordinarily and uncharacteristically focused—on killing"* (Lavergne 1997, 91). Whitman purchased a Bowie knife, binoculars, and food rations for his next—and last—trip to the tower. Seemingly, these concrete steps toward evil committed him to the crime. His depression, moreover, was such that he felt life unworthy of living. On August 1, shortly after midnight, Whitman killed his mother with a hunting knife. His delusional plan was to keep her from "suffering" after his own anticipated demise on the tower. Then, sometime after two o'clock that same morning, he stabbed his wife to death as she slept.

After coolly phoning his wife's employer (to say she'd not be coming in to work), cashing checks, and buying additional supplies, Charlie entered the tower at 11:35 a.m. Killing commenced as soon as he reached the observation deck on the twenty-eighth floor. En route to the deck, Charlie attacked any and all who got in his way. Afterward, his sniping began. He methodically shot people as they stood, walked, and conversed on the exposed flatland below. For many victims, the only danger signal received was the shock of a bullet piercing their body.

Finally, Austin police officers stormed the tower and shot Whitman dead at 1:24 p.m. Fourteen people were killed (plus two, his mother and wife, plus one, Whitman himself) and dozens more were wounded in what was then the largest simultaneous mass murder in U.S. history (Lavergne 1997).

In April 2006, I walked from my Austin Marriott hotel

room through the state capitol grounds to the University of Texas campus. There, looking up through stands of oak trees, I saw the fortresslike limestone tower. The UT Tower is still celebrated in artwork in stores and on walls around town. There was even a picture of it in my hotel room. In drawings the tower is impressive, but in person it has a chilling, ominous look. That April, I found no plaque commemorating Whitman's terrible deeds. As I walked around the UT Tower, I had a strong feeling Charlie knew he would never come down alive.

Before a murder takes place, telling changes show in the conduct, bearing, and emotional demeanor of the killer-to-be. A terrible decision has been made. The mind narrowly focuses and there is no turning back. As the body mobilizes to kill, body language changes. So could we have predicted that Charles Whitman would become such a murderer? I believe the answer is yes. Those who watched his behavior saw the warning signs:

- Physical abuse
- Weapons fancy
- Prior offenses
- Depression
- Chronic anger
- Spousal abuse
- Drug abuse
- Visible changes in demeanor

Taken together, these warning signs suggest a high probability of murder. The problem is our curious ability to overlook, disregard, and completely ignore them. As we'll see next, nowhere is our blindness to crime signals more dangerous than in the realm of spousal homicide.

KILLER IN THE MIST

Years before killing two by knife blade, one killer-to-be had already been arrested for violence. On January 1, 1989, he was apprehended at his posh home and later convicted of spousal battery. That New Year's Day, he admitted to officers that police had been called to his home on eight previous occasions (Lee 2002, 168).

In May 1993, at the California Beach Sushi restaurant in Hermosa Beach, a close friend observed as he exploded in terrible anger: "[His] face twitched uncontrollably. His body language was extremely aggressive. Horrified, I watched as sweat poured down his face. The veins in his neck bulged. His cheekbones bunched up, twitching beneath his skin" (Resnick 1994, 9). He was so angry at his ex-wife that, to maintain control, he followed her out of the restaurant and continued to fume, scream, and call her filthy names.

On October 25, 1993, there was another incident. The battered wife called 911 to report that her ex-husband was in the home after allegedly breaking down the back door to enter. In desperate tones, she begged for officers to save her. After still another incident of violence, in which the murderer-to-be picked up his victim and threw her against a wall, the woman kept photos of her injuries in a safe-deposit box to document her ex-husband's murderous potential.

On the foggy night of June 12, 1994, Nicole Brown Simpson, wearing a short black dress, was fatally slashed and stabbed on the walkway in front of her home. Earlier that evening, she had told O. J. Simpson that he could not have a custodial visit with his daughter, Sydney. O. J. complained to houseguest Kato Kaelin that his wife was now "playing hardball."

Nicole's companion, Ronald Goldman, wearing a light brown shirt and Levi's, was fatally stabbed as well. Los Angeles police found the pair lying in fresh pools of blood, Nicole on her walkway and Ron nearby. On the night of the double murder, according to Kato Kaelin, Nicole's ex-husband had on a dark sweat suit. A dark blue knit cap and bloodstained left-hand leather glove were found at the murder scene.

On February 4, 1997, after two lengthy court trials, Orenthal James "O. J." Simpson—the famous football player, sports announcer, and screen star—was found guilty of wrongful death for the murders by a civil court jury. O. J. was ordered to pay $8.5 million in compensatory and $25 million in punitive damages to the victims' families.

Prosecutors at the civil trial contended that O. J. had been stalking Nicole, and then killed her in a fit of rage. This is not atypical. In fact, crime statistics show that most men who kill their wives stalk them first. Stalking includes such behaviors as visual surveillance, pursuit, phone harassment, and sending unwanted gifts. Nicole accused O. J. of hiding in the bushes to spy on her. Kato Kaelin reported that O. J. had told him he'd peeped through her window while she had sex with another man.

> Stalking is a course of conduct directed at a specific person that would cause a reasonable person to feel fear. Almost 90% of stalkers are men.
> —National Center for the Victims of Crime

At his earlier, criminal trial, O. J. was acquitted on October 3, 1995. This was due in part to a clever trick he played with his hands. To see if the bloodstained glove was actually his, Simpson was asked to try it on. As forensic scientist Mark Benecke writes in his book *Murderous Methods*, "Because the defendant himself was to slip it over his hand, it was not hard for him to make it appear too narrow by stretching his thumb and his little finger apart as far as he could" (Benecke 2005, 181).

Simpson's clever trick was matched by his lawyer Johnnie Cochran's clever rhyme, "If the glove doesn't fit, you must acquit." Like the con man's swindle, O. J.'s criminal trial came down to theatrics, props, and sleight of hand. But could we have predicted that this international celebrity, O. J. Simpson, of all people, would become a murderer? Judging by these warning signs, the answer is yes:

- Episodic bursts of anger
- Controlling personality
- Tendency toward progressive violence
- Spousal abuse
- Stalking
- Acute triggering anger

A Chicago police officer not associated with the case said what most police officers know all too well: "With domestic murders, there's always a history of violence. It's very rare that somebody just goes off. You just don't go to the dresser and get the handgun and shoot your husband through the *Tribune*. That just isn't done. There's usually a *long* history of violence" (Fletcher 1991, 137; author's emphasis). O. J. trial prosecutor Scott Gordon put it more succinctly: "Simpson was killing Nicole for years—she finally died on June twelfth" (de Becker 1997, 173).

From a tape-recorded police interview on June 13, 1994— one day after the murders—O. J.'s voice sounded guilty to former

Los Angeles County prosecutor Vincent Bugliosi. "Most notable," he wrote, "there's a total absence of outrage and resentment, or even surprise on his part, that he's being considered a suspect in these murders" (Bugliosi 1996, 104).

TALE OF THE KNIT CAP

As the line of questioning changes in a courtroom, watch for coincident changes in nonverbal behavior. Recall how O. J. Simpson sat cryptically silent for nine months at his criminal murder trial. As O. J. listened to testimony about the location of his infamous dark blue knit cap, he protested—vigorously shook his head back and forth—against what he knew to be false. But as he listened to testimony accusing him of murdering his wife, Simpson showed no visible protest. Like Scott Peterson, he protested too little. Simpson remained motionless in his seat, casually doodling with a pen. Why the stark contrast in O. J.'s demeanor? You be the judge.

As Vincent Bugliosi later wrote, "No sound in any courtroom is as loud as the defendant's silence when he is accused of the most serious crime of all, murder, and he chooses not to deny it from the witness stand" (Bugliosi 1996, 25).

THE CASE OF THE MISSING EMOTIONS

In the cases of Charles Whitman and O. J. Simpson, telling emotions were visible in body language before the crimes. In the case of convicted double murderer Scott Peterson, there was little body language or evident emotion at all after the crime. As we saw in chapter 1, jurors commented that Peterson had seemed apathetic, indifferent, and unemotional throughout the trial. But how did he behave before the murder? What did his body language say about hidden emotion?

Emotion has deep, convoluted roots in animal nature. An emotion is a pleasant or unpleasant mental state organized in the brain's limbic system, in what neurologists call the "old mammalian brain." These ancient brain regions, which lie beneath centers for conscious thought in gray matter above, animate all our feelings and moods. Emotions are mammalian elaborations of vertebrate arousal patterns, in which neurochemicals such as dopamine, noradrenaline, and serotonin step up or step down the brain's activity level.

Since they are visible in body movements, we can see and read each other's emotions with relative ease. We can detect and decipher clear feelings of agreement, anger, certainty, control, disagreement, disgust, disliking, embarrassment, fear, happiness, hate, interest, liking, love, sadness, shame, surprise, and uncertainty. Each is expressed apart from words.

If a suspect masks his feelings or seems to feel nothing at all, a message is nonetheless sent. As anthropologist Ray Birdwhistell—who was the founder of kinesics, the scientific study of body language—taught, "You cannot not behave." An absence of gestures can tell as much about emotion as gestures themselves.

Prior to Scott Peterson's killings, according to family members, he and his wife, Laci, had been the "perfect couple." But Scott changed when Laci became pregnant with their first child. He told Laci he would not welcome a baby into his life. "He said he didn't want to have children," Laci tearfully told her mother (Rocha 2006, 57).

On November 20, 2002, at the Elephant Bar in Fresno, California, Peterson had his first face-to-face meeting with Amber Frey, who would soon be his girlfriend. The couple went to a Japanese restaurant for dinner that night. Peterson, the married man who lived in Modesto and worked as a fertilizer salesman, told Frey grandiose lies—that he lived alone in a big house in

Sacramento, and had a career that took him "all over the world— from Cairo to Paris" (Frey 2005, 6). They had sexual relations on this, their first date.

Scott's behavior changed. His half sister, Anne Bird, noted a definite shift in her half brother's demeanor. On a late-November 2002 family trip to Disneyland, while pregnant Laci seemed happy, Anne noticed that Scott seemed distant and "strangely subdued." He spent a good deal of time on his cell phone and paid little attention to his wife or family.

Anne Bird saw another odd sign on the Disneyland trip. Scott kept his head down. A moment of family panic had spread through Anne's fourth-floor hotel room when she noticed her three-year-old son was missing. But in the momentary chaos until they found him, Scott stayed coolly on his cell phone and "never even looked up."

Later, at Laci's baby shower on December 10, 2002, Anne noticed that Scott was once more subdued, "not quite himself again." Before Laci's murder, telling changes showed in Scott's conduct, bearing, and emotional demeanor. A terrible decision may already have been made. As the body mobilizes to kill, body language changes.

But how could a man even think about killing his pregnant wife? Answers to this question came on March 21, 2001, nearly two years before the Peterson murders. A prophetic study was published in the prestigious *Journal of the American Medical Association*. In their article "Enhanced Surveillance for Pregnancy-Associated Mortality, Maryland 1993–1998," Diana Cheng and Isabelle Horon opened the door on a previously unknown brand of murder. They discovered that the leading cause of death among pregnant women was homicide.

In what later was found to be a nationwide pattern, men kill their pregnant partners to keep from paying child support, from damaging their careers, and from being tied down—generally, in other words, to protect and maintain their freedom. Pat Brown, a criminal profiler and president of the Sexual Homicide Exchange in Minneapolis, tells women to watch for four warning signs. Be cautious about becoming pregnant with men who (1) lack concern for your happiness and well-being, (2) are manipulative, (3) exhibit grandiose thinking, and (4) have a history of dishonesty.

Laci Peterson was murdered on December 23 or 24, 2002. In the most likely scenario, she was drowned in her own back-yard swimming pool, then hidden in Scott's recently purchased aluminum fishing boat, and finally dropped into San Francisco Bay tied to concrete weights made by Peterson earlier for that purpose.

On April 14, 2003, Laci's body washed ashore one day after her son's body was found on the same shoreline, near Richmond, California. Could we have predicted that mild-mannered Scott Peterson, who showed neither Charles Whitman's weapons fancy nor O. J. Simpson's outbursts of rage, was capable of first-degree murder? Based on his nonverbal signals before the crime, the probable answer is yes:

- Manipulative charmer
- Grandiosity
- Chronic, aggressive liar
- Obsessive fear of losing freedom
- Acute sexual infatuation with another woman

RECOGNIZING FACES

One of the first steps in a murder investigation is searching for eyewitnesses at the crime scene. For an eyewitness, the most easily identified body part is the suspect's face. The face is every human's personal signature and exclusive trademark.

With switchblade-inflicted jagged scars running down the right side of his face, Al Capone was an easy man to identify. Capone, a gangster from Chicago in the 1920s and 1930s, allegedly masterminded the 1929 St. Valentine's Day Massacre in which seven rival gang members were killed. "Scarface" Al's visage was easily described in words.

Most faces are not so easily captured by verbal labels. Our brain's innate ability to recognize a murder suspect's face far exceeds that of any spoken language to describe it. Dedicated areas in the brain's temporal lobes enable us to pick out the faces we've seen at crime scenes. But since we lack a sufficient vocabulary of specialized "face" words, our ability to describe faces linguistically is poor. Identity clues used by the Chicago police consist only of general, all-purpose words such as high, low, wide, and narrow foreheads; smooth, creased, and wrinkled skin; long, wide, flat, pug, and Roman noses; wide, narrow, and flared nostrils; sunken, filled-out, dried, oily, and wrinkled cheeks; prominent, high, low, wide, and fleshy cheekbones; corners turned up, down, and level for the mouth; thin, medium, and full upper and lower lips; double chin, protruding Adam's apple, and hanging jowls for necks; and round, oval, pointed, square, small, and double chins.

For the human observer, facial recognition is more art than science. In 2002, police in Baltimore learned that the murder suspect a witness had picked from a photo lineup had actually died a year before the murder was committed (Levesque 2003). In their book *Mistaken Identification*, Brian Cutler and Steven Penrod estimate that for every million convictions in the U.S., five thousand are misidentified and are thus convicted wrongfully (Cutler and Penrod 1995, 3).

Recognizing faces from ethnic or racial groups other than your own can be especially challenging. Research on the so-called cross-race effect, a misnamed but well-studied phenomenon, finds that black witnesses are 50 percent more likely to misidentify white suspects, and white witnesses are 50 percent more likely to misidentify black suspects, because "they all look alike" (see, e.g., MacLin and Malpass 2001). In part, says neuroscientist Scania de Schonen of René Descartes University in Paris, this is because human beings develop face-recognition skills at an early age, from around birth to nine. Since a white child develops an eye for familial white faces, in adulthood he or she may be less able to identify African American, Asian, or Middle Eastern faces in a lineup.

In hindsight, a classic example of the cross-race effect may have occurred in the famous "Quincy Five" murder case of 1971. Five white eyewitnesses wrongly identified five African American men as perpetrators in the murder of Deputy Sheriff Khomas Revels in Tallahassee, Florida. "All of the men were later exonerated when the *three* actual perpetrators were found" (Natarajan 2003). More than racial prejudice may have been in the witnesses' eyes. There may also have been anger and subliminal fear. Recent evidence suggests that greater activation of the brain's fear center, the amygdala, takes place when one views faces from a racial or ethnic out-group than when viewing faces from one's own racial in-group (Anonymous 2000a). Facial *un*familiarity, it appears, can breed contempt.

Iowa State University psychologist Gary L. Wells, an expert in identification issues, recommends that police videotape witnesses at lineups so jurors can see how confident they are in identifying the suspects they pick. The problem with lineups, generally, is that witnesses tend to select an individual who looks more like the perpetrator than others in the line. He or she may not look exactly like the perpetrator, but through a process of elimination, an eyewitness tends to identify someone as the group's most likely suspect.

Since police officers who know the perpetrator's identity can unwittingly influence witnesses, Wells suggests using "double-blind" lineups in which officers don't know who in the assembled group are the suspects.

To minimize cases of mistaken identity in the traditional "serial" lineup, Minnesota police have experimented with lineups that are "sequential." Their data show that viewing murder suspects individually—one by one rather than all together in a group—substantially reduces incorrect IDs.

THE FACE OF A MURDERER

Facial recognition is the act of identifying a face that has been seen before. Recognition is the awareness of having seen, met, known—or known of—another by recalling the distinctive features of his or her face. The ability to recognize and recall thousands of faces easily at a glance is a unique talent possessed by human beings alone. Studies show that as our eyes scan faces, they make repeated rest stops at the lips and eyes. Viewed from the side, our eyes hover about the profiled nose, eye, ear, and lips. Facial recognition is an active process that leads us to see faces even where there are none, as in clouds, rock formations, screen doors, and shrouds, and even on the surface of the moon.

In Victorian times, many believed that a murderer's face would be indelibly imprinted upon the victim's eyes as a recognizable image. If only this were true, police would not need physical descriptions, lineups, or mug shots to catch a killer. Electronic aids in use today, such as closed-circuit cameras and facial-recognition software, are helpful, but there's still no substitute for seeing a face in person. For purposes of identification and protection from harm, we need to look at facial features and watch their movements.

A murderer's face telegraphs menace not in physiognomy but in expressive motions or equally expressive immobility. Each has a tale to tell. Suspicion was raised when O. J. Simpson's face went ballistic at the California Beach Sushi, and when Scott Peterson's face went blank in court. Both facial expressions were unusual, aberrant, and anomalous; both, therefore, were meaningful. In the context of killing, each signaled beyond a doubt that something terribly wrong was about to happen or already had. The something, of course, was murder. Two innocent women died at the hands of two bad men. While both men lied, their own bodies spoke the truth.

Crime signals are visible warning signs that show someone has broken, or is about to break, the law. Murderers, whether violent ones like the Texas sniper or devious ones like Scott Peterson, emit telling cues before their misdeeds. Not all of their victims, however, see, read, or heed the signs.

Thomas Eckman was a clock tower victim standing on the ground. Whitman shot him dead from on high without warning. Eckman saw nothing of Charlie, the man, before he fired the shot. Laci Peterson must have felt something was wrong with Scott, but may not have read danger in his furtive demeanor. Nicole Simpson read danger in O. J.'s aggressive body, but did not fully take heed. Neither, apparently, did the police.

When someone's behavior seems unusual—"creepy," "unusually quiet," "extremely aggressive," or "strangely subdued"—trust the signal. Should the person's nonverbal signs suggest potential for harm, prepare for the possibility. As you've seen, crime signals vary quite widely. There's no surefire formula. That said, here are several warning signs to be especially alert to:

- History of physical violence or spousal abuse
- Weapons fancy
- Episodic bursts of rage
- Stalking
- Grandiosity and dishonesty
- Manipulative personality
- Acute triggering anger

In the next chapter, you will learn to read the warning signs of imminent assault. What does body language look like before a physical attack? Again, we draw from the world of real crime.

5

PRELUDE TO AN ASSAULT

Dundy jumped up and tapped Spade's chest with the ends of two bent fingers. "Keep your God-damned paws off me."

—SAM SPADE to San Francisco police lieutenant Dundy *The Maltese Falcon*

THE CRIMINAL WORLD is a dangerous place. Physical attack may come suddenly. But are there warnings?

While walking with my wife on a crowded sidewalk in Bologna, Italy, a tall, dark-haired young man approached me from the front. Suddenly, without any warning, he raised his right hand and poked a stiffened index finger firmly on my chest. There was no time to react. Had it been a knife or loaded gun, I might not be here today.

Bologna is not a tourist town. But my wife's blue eyes and blond hair may have marked us as tourists. Perhaps I was a likely victim for panhandling. We'll never know. The man just looked into my eyes, thumped my chest, and went on his way down the street.

While robbing a tavern in Chicago, Illinois, a short young man with a smooth, boyish face ordered the owner, a waiter, and a customer to raise their hands. Then suddenly, and seemingly without warning, the man known as Baby Face Nelson shot and killed the patron with a single shotgun blast to his chest.

Thankfully, the other two were spared. But why did Baby Face Nelson kill the customer? A clue was the expression on the latter's face. Unlike the owner or waiter, the customer, a stockbroker named Edwin Thompson, had smiled a nervous grin. In assaultive situations, a grinning face can show or suggest mockery. "Don't smile, you," Baby Face growled as he fatally pulled the trigger (Burrough 2004, 104).

In these two cases, one amusing, the other deadly serious, there was no warning sign prior to an aggressive act. The gun, of course, was a clue, yet there was no telling who would be shot. Baby Face Nelson was known to have enjoyed killing, more than his fellow Depression-era gangster peers. Showing no obvious sign beforehand, Nelson was like the North American grizzly bear (*Ursus arctos horribilis*), one of a handful of animals known to attack without warning. Most animals—humans included—telegraph that they are about to assail before assailing.

From chapter 4, recall Faye Resnick's description of O. J. Simpson's rage at Nicole Brown in the California Beach Sushi café: "Horrified, I watched as sweat poured down his face. The veins in his neck bulged. His cheekbones bunched up, twitching beneath his skin" (Resnick 1994, 9). In response to O. J.'s rant, Nicole's face became rigid with fear. Verbally, Nicole raised her voice to exclaim, "I'm afraid of you when you're like this!" (Resnick 1994, 11).

As the brain mobilizes for attack, physiological arousal shows throughout the body. What Faye Resnick saw in O. J.'s face is quite common: sweat surfaces on the skin, blood vessels pulsate, and jaws clench. Each of these cues is a declarative signal that the nervous system has been dangerously aroused. Shown in a context of anger, these cues could be vital warning signs.

SKIN SIGNALS

Unless one is sunbathing, exercising, or nursing a fever, the face should be relatively dry. Otherwise, if you see moisture glistening on another's forehead or temples, above the upper lip, or around the ears, ask yourself, "Why?" In chapter 1, we saw with Sherlock Holmes that facial sweat may be read as a sign of deception. But in an angry encounter, facial sweating may be read as another kind of sign, one showing that the anger at hand is getting out of hand.

You may wonder how a sweaty forehead could signal both aggression and deceit. It's because the sweat-gland cells that discharge their watery or eccrine perspiration are linked to the same nerve fibers. Basically, skin sweats whether you are on the attack, or fearful of being attacked for telling a lie. Whether fighting or fleeing, a sweaty face looks the same. In either, sweat on the brow or above the upper lip spells arousal.

In tandem with facial sweat, you should watch a face for its color. Like sweat beads around the mouth, sudden facial pallor or rapid reddening may signal stepped-up visceral feelings and emotions of the fight-or-flight response.

Fight or flight is an ancient sympathetic-nervous-system response. For our primeval aquatic ancestors, the jawed fishes, accelerated heartbeat, raised blood sugar, and hormones released from the adrenal gland prepared an alarmed fish to chase and bite or turn tail and flee. Today, our adrenal glands work the same way.

Pallor associated with rage shows through constriction of tiny blood vessels near the surface of the face. The pale, ashen skin tone is brought on by the release of large amounts of two hormones, adrenaline and noradrenaline. Associated with embarrassment or slight to moderate anger, a flushed face—which may commence with faint blushing atop the ears—is caused by dilation of blood vessels prompted by a single hormone, adrenaline. At present, physiological differences between fear and anger are not well understood, but seeing a shift from redness to paleness in a face is definitely cause for alarm.

PULSATING ARTERIES

When Faye Resnick watched the "veins" in O. J.'s neck bulge, she really meant arteries. Both veins and arteries are hollow conducting tubes, but they differ in structure and function. Since veins drain blood back to the heart from the body, they are thinner and do not pulsate. Thus, veins have little to "say" about potentially murderous feelings and moods.

Arteries, on the other hand, speak volumes. Since they work with the heart to push blood upward and downward—out of the heart into the body—they have thicker walls with muscular lining. Artery muscles contract and visibly pulsate. In extreme anger or rage, the swelling pulsations stand out clearly on one's face and neck. The most obvious throbbing can be seen in the neck area below the earlobes, where the prominent carotid artery speaks its mind. When carotids beckon, police and customs officers heed their call. Someone may have something to hide.

Less visible but equally telling is the web of smaller arteries that branch upward into the face from the carotid below. When feelings run high, facial arteries pulsate at the back of the lower jaw (the facial artery itself), in the temple area immediately in front of the ear (the superficial temporal artery), above and below the lips (superior and inferior labial arteries), beside the nose (angular artery), at the cheekbones (transverse facial artery), and in the middle of the forehead running vertically above the eyebrows (supraorbital artery).

Though anatomically complex, facial arteries are easy to read. As someone mobilizes for combat, these blood vessels mark the face like a pulsing red rash. Noticeable facial arteries in someone who seems "merely angry" can reveal the onset of potentially dangerous rage—someone who's now "really angry."

A DISARMING SHOULDER SHRUG

Most signals in this chapter telegraph danger, but a few suggest safety. In the context of anger, the most reassuring of our "safe" facial expressions, gestures, and postures come from the shoulder-shrug display. As a rule, a person who shrugs telegraphs that he's in no mood to fight.

In 1872, Charles Darwin identified a global body-movement pattern called the shrug display. The display is an interrelated set of ten body motions, ranging from the head to the toes, which is used worldwide to show psychological helplessness, resignation, and uncertainty.

Individually or in combination, nonverbal signs from the shrug display—including sideward head tilts, elevated shoulders, and pigeon toes—suggest feelings of resignation, powerlessness, and submission. Since they show that a person is not likely to attack, seeing shrug-related signs in someone—especially in a person who seems angry or upset—is good news. The shrug display involves the entire body in a defensive, protective crouch. As originally described by Darwin, the display consists of (1) raised or lifted shoulders (recall the Brad Jackson case in chapter 2), (2) a head tilt sideward, (3) elbows bent and tucked into the sides of the body, (4) reaching out with an open and upraised palm, (5) lifted eyebrows, and (6) an opened mouth. A century later, (7) pouted lips, (8) knock-knees, (9) bowing forward at the waist, and (10) pigeon toes (toes angled in) were added to the display (Givens 1977).

The shoulder-shrug display originates from a crouching posture, a primordial self-protective stance brought on by the tactile-withdrawal reflex. We automatically cower from unwelcome touches to our skin. In a social setting, we cower from aggressive people looking to do us harm. Submissive feelings find expression in coordinated muscle contractions designed to bend, flex, and simultaneously rotate diverse body parts, to visually "shrink" the frame and show a harmless "lower" profile. Since body motions of the shrug were designed for self-protection—for defense rather than offense—they suggest that one is more likely to flee than fight.

BITING COMMENTARY

"His cheekbones bunched up, twitching beneath his skin." In this case, Resnick's description was anatomically correct. You can feel the jaw's bunching with your fingertips. Palpate your upper cheek area as you clench your teeth. The bony movements you feel, near where the lower jaw connects to the skull above, is a visible sign of biting. In biting, the jaws close tightly to cut, grip, grasp, or tear with the teeth. We bite to chew, to clench the jaws in anger and frustration, or to inflict pain. Our animal nature clearly shows in the eagerness with which we bite our enemies.

In New York City, 1,500 people report being bitten by another human each year—five times the reported figure for rat bites.

In both rats and humans, a bite's prime mover is the masseter muscle. Like the muscles of facial expression, which enable us to smile or frown based on the emotions we feel, the masseter is highly excitable. It is controlled by the trigeminal nerve (cranial V). Since the trigeminal is an emotionally sensitive special visceral nerve, strong anger may cause the jaw muscles to contract in uncontrollable biting movements. Nonverbally, at the California Beach Sushi restaurant, O. J. was in a biting mood.

JAWS OUT OF CONTROL

Along with their role in chewing and eating, our remote ancestors' jaws, teeth, and jaw muscles played a defensive role: the face was used as a weapon. This is dramatically the case today in crocodiles, gorillas, grizzly bears—and human beings.

On June 28, 1997, in a televised boxing match, heavyweight fighter "Iron" Mike Tyson committed a major foul by biting off a one-inch piece of Evander Holyfield's right ear and spitting it onto the floor of the ring. Two points were deducted from his score, but in the third round Tyson tried to bite Holyfield's left ear and was disqualified from the competition. Clearly, Tyson had used his face as a weapon.

On May 28, 1981, I interviewed counselor Janis Goodman at Northwest Center for the Retarded in Seattle, Washington, about a minor biting incident that happened just outside her office. I entered the room through its narrow doorway—the only way in or out. Janis's desk was to my immediate left, and a couch for visitors was in the very back, facing the doorway about ten feet away.

Janis well remembered the incident. When one is attacked, time stands still and details leave indelible impressions on the mind. Her scheduled meeting with "Leo," a large twenty-five-year-old male client, began when he entered her office, walked to the back, and sat down on the couch.

Leo seemed "agitated," Janis said. She noted he had run, not walked, to her office. He turned his face away to the side as she talked to him, and wouldn't say a word to her. This is another instance of cutoff, a form of gaze avoidance in which the head turns fully away to one side. Leo's sustained cutoff revealed strong disliking.

When Janis brought up his "problem behavior," the purpose of the meeting, Leo turned his face toward her, abruptly stood up, walked quickly to her desk, got physically close, and beat the air above her head with his fists, a signal pregnant with meaning.

In the context of anger, showing a clenched fist is a universal sign of aggression. A fist is a gesture made with the hand closed, the fingers flexed, and the tactile pads held firmly against the palm. A tightly closed fist signals an aroused emotional state, as in anger, excitement (e.g., to cheer on a team), or fear. In Pakistan, displaying a fist toward another is an "obscene insult" (Morris 1994, 71). Politicians who have used the aggressive fist gesture to hammer home rhetorical points include Adolf Hitler, Nikita Khrushchev, and Manuel Noriega (Blum 1988).

In nursery school children, the beating movement "is an overarm blow with the palm side of the lightly clenched fist. The arm is sharply bent at the elbow and raised to a vertical position then brought down with great force on the opponent, hitting any part of him that gets in the way" (Blurton Jones 1967, 355). Children born blind and deaf innately clench their fists in anger (Eibl-Eibesfeldt 1971, 12). As behavioral biologist Desmond Morris attests, the closed fist is a worldwide sign used to show forceful emphasis and threat (Morris 1994, 70, 72–73).

> That's what makes a blow from the hand, Flask, fifty times more savage
> to bear than a blow from a cane. The living member—that
> makes the living insult, my little man.
> —Herman Melville, *Moby-Dick*

Janis went on to describe Leo's "large eyes," closed mouth, tense lips, and "frown." He made no vocalizations or any sound at all. After beating the air with fisted hands, he turned, walked back, and sat again on the couch. As we'll see later in this chapter, physical assaults are often preceded by momentary silence.

Next, Leo's girlfriend, "Myra," came into the office and sat next to him on the couch. Empowered by each other's presence, they started yelling at Janis. Biologists call this "ritualized mobbing" or "to aggression out." By aggressing in tandem at Janis, they felt closer as a pair. Feeling her gang of two's anger, Janis backed up and stood in the doorway. Leo and Myra then got up and made a beeline for the door. On the way out, Leo grabbed Janis's wrists, shook them, and pushed her into a drinking fountain inset in the wall.

Janis hit her hip on the hallway wall and became pinned against it and the fountain. Then, topping off his aggressive display, Leo grabbed Janis's arm, bit her forearm through her corduroy jacket and blouse, and hung on with his teeth for "a second or two." Afterward, he let her go and fled down the hall. In the end, the physical damage to Janis was relatively minor, but the psychic damage of Leo's bite remained for years. It was more insult, nonverbally, than injury.

This case illustrates a principle that is as true today as it was millions of years ago: The quickest way to aggression is to block an escape route. When cornered by a much larger cat, even a mouse will bite. Biologists call this the principle of "critical distance." Every animal, including *Homo sapiens*, has a specific distance at which, when another comes too close or blocks an escape route, it attacks on instinct. When Janis inadvertently blocked the doorway, Leo's face became his weapon. Had he had a knife or loaded gun, Janis might not be here today.

"When an animal has no escape route," French veterinarian Claude Beata observes, "to cross the virtual line called 'critical distance' . . . will trigger a sudden attack combining elements of fear, autonomous reactions and very violent sequences of aggressiveness. The bites will be without control, there is no warning phase but an explosion of violence and the induced wounds are severe with loss of tissue" (Beata 2001). Though not severely wounded, the fear Janis felt gripped in Leo's jaws was understandably intense.

Attacks with jaws and teeth may be symptomatic of intermittent explosive disorder, or IED. IED is an acute psychiatric illness characterized by episodes of violent outbursts of hostility, such as impulsively throwing or breaking objects, or physically attacking people. A study reported in the June 2006 edition of *Archives of General Psychiatry* estimated that as many as sixteen million Americans may be afflicted with IED. IED can swiftly escalate from damaging inanimate objects to harming human beings. There may be a sequential chain of events leading from object to person to lethal encounter. At the first sign of IED, break the chain and carefully walk away.

In psychology, a "behavioral chain" is a series of related acts, each of which reinforces and provides a trigger for what comes next. On October 1, 2006, nineteen-year-old "Josh" exploded in anger at his girlfriend, "Rachel," twenty, in the confines of her small Spokane apartment. After he slashed her leather chairs with a kitchen knife and kicked her TV through a window—object incidents—Rachel should have walked away. Unfortunately, she stayed, and Josh predictably escalated from attacking furniture to attacking his girlfriend. He threw Rachel against a wall, bloodied her nose, and bit her shoulder.

According to neighbors, Josh then pushed Rachel into a car, grabbed the young woman's hair to prevent her escape, and drove off. His kidnapped girlfriend finally managed to jump out of the moving vehicle. Had she not escaped, who knows what might have come next in the behavioral chain? A likely next step would have been a severe beating, or worse. She could have been killed. On December 9, 2006, Josh pleaded guilty to unlawful imprisonment and second-degree malicious mischief, and was sentenced to ninety days in jail.

LAWN RAGE

In the crime world, disputes over space and territory may quickly ignite into violence. An obvious example is road rage, in which seemingly minor affronts to right-of-way can lead to major rows on the highway. Human beings are very territorial creatures, and crossing invisible borders only invites aggression. The prime directive of personal space is that we may not come and go everywhere as we please. There are cultural rules and biological boundaries—explicit as well as subtle limits—to observe everywhere.

Scientific research on how we communicate in personal and public spaces began with studies of animal territoriality in the nineteenth and early twentieth centuries. In 1959, anthropologist Edward Hall popularized spatial research on human beings—calling it "proxemics"—in his classic book, *The Silent Language*. According to Hall, proxemics is the study of humankind's "perception and use of space." Since crossing invisible boundary lines may spark aggression, proxemic crime signals merit your closest attention.

"I just killed a kid," Charles Martin told the 911 operator. "I shot him with a goddamn 410 shotgun twice" (Borger 2006). On March 19, 2006, Martin, sixty-six, shot and killed his fifteen-year-old neighbor, Larry Mugrage, for the offense of walking across the senior citizen's well-groomed lawn. According to police reports, Martin first fired from his own house, then walked up to the boy's wounded body and fired at virtually point-blank range. Leaving the dead body where it lay on the teenager's front lawn, the alleged shooter calmly returned home and dialed 911.

Signs of Charles Martin's "lawn rage" had been evident for some time to the man's Union Township, Ohio, neighbors. Neighbors described Martin as a quiet man who lived alone. He had a habit of sitting outside, beneath the U.S. and Navy flags he flew, quietly enjoying his neat lawn. Though well liked in the neighborhood, Martin reportedly displayed explosive rage should neighbors walk on his lawn or mow across the invisible boundary line separating his turf from theirs. As one neighbor recalled, "He was really warped on that stuff" (Borger 2006). On April 26, 2007, a jury found Charles Martin guilty of killing neighbor Larry Mugrage.

> Damn, I poured my whole life into this lawn, my heart, my soul, the tender feelings I've held back from my family. . . . Look, some people hoist a flag to show they love their country. Well, my lawn is my flag.
> —Hank Hill, *King of the Hill* (quoted in the *Spokane [Wash.] Spokesman-Review*, May 28, 2000)

The territorial sense of the word "lawn" traces to its ancient Indo-European root, *lendh*–, "open land." A lawn, according to

The Nonverbal Dictionary, is "a plot of carefully groomed grass, and any of several decorative artifacts (e.g., white pickets or plastic pink flamingos) placed upon its surface" (Givens 2003). Semiotically, lawns are more than gardens. They communicate, mark territory, and betoken social status. Their dimensions and decor define the yard space and provide tangible evidence that "this land is mine."

Prior to the shooting, Martin and Mugrage had reportedly exchanged words. But in this case, the fighting words were less incendiary than the boy's nonverbal act of stepping across a border. Had Mugrage understood the irrational depth of Martin's lawn rage, he might have chosen a safer route. Though often invisible, boundaries are psychologically real. The territorial roots of road rage and lawn rage are one and the same.

COMBATIVE EYES

From the December 19, 1969, edition of *Life* magazine, the face of Charles Manson stares out evilly from the cover. His eyes are reminiscent of the Dracula movies of 1931, 1973, and 1979, in which actors Bela Lugosi, Jack Palance, and Frank Langella consciously widened their eyes before biting a victim's neck to draw blood.

In this, the most widely publicized photo of the convicted mass murderer, celebrity killer, and leader of the infamous 1960s gang known as the Manson Family, we see little more than Manson's wide, riveting eyes. You see white showing above the right eye's iris, and the entire upper half of his left iris shows beneath his upper eyelid. Eyes like his just aren't "normal."

In its normal alert-and-resting position, the lower eyelid barely touches, or covers less than a fourth of the bottom circumference of our iris, while the upper eyelid covers one-third to one-half of its top. When excited, we widen our eye openings, and we narrow them when we feel threatened. Sudden eyelid closure is part of a protective, mammalian facial grimace brought on by the startle reflex. Suddenly widened eyes reflect emotions of the fight-or-flight response.

Like the wide eyes of actors playing Dracula, Charles Manson's *Life* magazine eyes are deliberately wide open. Manson opened them on purpose to mug for the camera, to make a face for effect. We know this because, as in the alert-and-resting position, his lower lids rise to partially cover the bottom circumferences of his irises.

Though evil-looking in his photo, Manson's eyes are not combative. He does not look poised for attack. Had his eyes been fully widened, with white showing all around, above and below his irises, there would have been cause for alarm. Had he shown what I call "flashbulb eyes," it would have been prudent to take cover.

Flashbulb eyes are an involuntary, dramatic enlargement of both eyes, performed in situations of very high emotion, such as intense anger or terror. Maximal opening of the eyelids takes place to show the eyeballs' roundness, curvature, and protrusion. When we are truly angry, rather than feigning the emotion for effect in a conversation, two involuntary visceral muscles in the eyelids—called superior and inferior tarsals—widen the eye slits to make eyeballs appear noticeably bigger, rounder, and whiter.

Like another visceral sign of emotion, dilated pupils, flashbulb eyes are controlled by impulses from the nervous system's fight-or-flight division, working through the spinal cord's superior cervical ganglion. As visceral signs, true flashbulb eyes are difficult to produce on purpose or at will. Thus, they are all the more trustworthy as nonverbal cues, especially of terror or rage.

In an angry man or woman, flashbulb eyes can be decoded as a danger sign of imminent physical attack.

PUGNACIOUS PUPILS

In *Life* magazine's December 19, 1969, cover photo of Charles Manson, we see pupils that are safely small and constricted. The good news here is that his sympathetic nervous system seems to be in a quiet or paused mode. He is seemingly calm and semirelaxed. Had they been significantly enlarged or dilated, we would see a man ominously on alert, coiled and ready for action. In constriction, rest-and-digest nerve fibers activate the pupillary sphincter muscles of the irises to shrink the pupils. In dilation, fight-or-flight nerve fibers from the superior cervical ganglion activate dilator muscles to expand the diameter of the pupils. When someone seems angry, enlarged pupils can signal pugnacious pique.

BELLIGERENT BLINKING

When the going gets tough, the eyelids get going. Our blink rate reflects psychological arousal in the manner of a polygraph test. The normal, resting blink rate of a human being is twenty closures per minute, with the average blink lasting one-quarter of a second (Karson 1992). Significantly higher rates may reflect emotional stress as aroused by the fight-or-flight response.

Boston College psychologist Joseph J. Tecce has studied blinking in the fiercely competitive arena of U.S. presidential politics. Candidates for the president's job engage in face-to-face duels for votes, in verbal contests called televised debates. In the 1996 presidential debates, candidate Bob Dole averaged 147 blinks per minute—seven times above normal. President Bill

Clinton averaged 99 blinks a minute, reaching 117 when asked about increases in teen drug use, a sensitive issue of the day (Smith 1996). In general, the average blinking rate for someone speaking on TV is 31 to 50 blinks a minute—twice the relaxed rate.

We blink faster when our nervous system is excited and slower when it's calm. Eyelid movements reflect bodily arousal levels established in our primitive hindbrain, the evolutionary old brain area located at the base of our skull. The specific mechanism is the hindbrain's reticular activating system, or RAS. Emotion from the limbic system stimulates the RAS to release an excitatory chemical, dopamine, into ancient vision centers of the midbrain above.

We bat our eyelids faster before launching into a fight as well as before fleeing from one.

"Eye blinking is another well-known primate movement," biologist Niko Tinbergen told *Psychology Today* magazine. "The moment you have the least little bit of stress, the eyelids blink, bang! bang! bang!" When you see rapid blinking in someone who seems upset or angry, it's time to take a step backward, beyond harm's reach.

BELLICOSE BREATHING

Along with assault warnings afforded by facial sweating, skin color, pulsing arteries, biting movements, flashbulb eyes, and rapid blinking, visible and audible changes take place in the way we breathe. Prompted by strongly felt emotion, an increase in breathing rate takes place. Nerve cells in the brain's hypothalamus tell respiratory centers to speed up. More oxygen is needed to fuel the impending fight, or to fuel retreat from harm's way.

Breathing is visible because when you inhale, the diaphragm and muscles between ribs contract to enlarge the chest. When you exhale, these muscles relax and your chest cavity gets smaller. The cycle repeats with each breath. In an angry situation, take heed should someone's breathing rate noticeably increase.

SILENCE IN SEATTLE

In a study of assault warnings I did in Seattle, Washington, with the cooperation of the United States District Court, the FBI, the Seattle Police Department, and other agencies, I learned that one of the most commonly recognized danger signs is silence.

Silence is the condition or quality of being difficult or impossible to hear, as in walking stealthily, swallowing a cry, curtailing bodily noises, and refraining from speech. Synonyms for silent include "secretive," "reserved," and "tight-lipped." The last in particular implies a conscious decision to withhold information.

Animals from reptiles to human beings have devised ingenious means to be silent in order to avoid detection. In an August 27, 2001, *USA Today* editorial—"Silence Speaks Volumes"—U.S. representative Gary Condit was criticized for his tight-lipped refusal to discuss his relationship with House intern Chandra Levy, in connection with her mysterious disappearance. Reserving the biological right to remain silent, Condit said nothing.

If silence is golden, it is also manipulative, and a sign that something bad is about to happen or be revealed.

In a typical attack scenario from my field notes, Seattle police responded to neighbors who heard gunshots outside. Two men had been shooting rabbits in their backyard with a hunting rifle. Officers arrived and knocked on the front door, and one of the men answered.

Officers Byers and Hamlet entered the men's living room to discuss the shooting. Officer Hamlet described the man who let them in as "hostile, bitter, and down on whites." Then the second man walked down the stairs—silently, according to both officers—entered the living room, and sat on the couch. Hamlet, who was standing six to ten feet away, described him as "seemingly upset" but verbally silent.

Then suddenly, "without warning," the seated man stood, rushed in "two steps," and "lunged" toward Hamlet, grabbing his badge. As he charged, he gave the officer direct eye contact and yelled, "Get out! Get out of my house!" Hamlet reacted by punching the man's mouth with his fist. The officer showed me the tooth scar still on his hand.

Officer Hamlet said he'd felt something was wrong because the man descended the staircase in silence. Like a stalking tiger, he made no warning sound whatsoever, and then kept silent on the couch. As with other attacks noted in my Seattle report, this one came suddenly, in silence, from a seemingly dormant, quiescent body. Like facial sweating, pulsing arteries, and flashbulb eyes, inappropriate silence can signal that the mind and body are mobilizing to fight.

Officer Gary Vargas of the Washington State Parole Office detailed just such a case, a home visit with a twenty-one-year-old parolee named "Tom." Tom stared at the officer with big, wide-open eyes, and Vargas noticed sweat on the young man's brow. Gradually the parolee backed off, retreated, and silently sat down on the living room couch. His demeanor had become passive, his head and upper body leaned forward, and he avoided the officer's gaze.

Vargas noticed the man begin to scoot along the couch toward the mantel, upon which lay a pair of sharp scissors. All of a sudden, the quiet young man stood up, yelled, grabbed the scissors, and put the blades to his own throat. Suspecting Tom was on drugs, Vargas backed away, and, as if on cue, the scissors dropped to the floor. By stepping backward, Vargas had reassured the man that his critical distance would not be invaded. The self-inflicted aggression ceased as suddenly as it had begun.

Fear can quickly change into aggression, and vice versa. Police officers are trained to disarm aggressors psychologically and physically, but the rest of us should simply back away. Like storm warnings, an assault warning tells you to prepare for the worst. Some of the warnings we've discussed include:

- Facial sweat in the context of anger
- Sudden shifts from flushed skin to pallor
- Pulsating carotid and facial arteries
- Tightly clenched jaw muscles
- Silence after a rage
- Tightly fisted hands
- Rapid blinking
- Flashbulb eyes

In his classic book *Officer Down, Code Three* (1976), Pierce Brooks gives sound advice: Watch the hands and palms. Since hands are prime movers in fighting, holding weapons, and concealing them, your attention should always be on fingers, hands, and palms.

The preparatory-intention movements of these organs can reveal that an assault is about to happen before it begins.

In the next chapter, you will learn to decipher the body language of a different breed of offenders, those who prey on people of all ages, but especially the very young.

6

THE PREDATORY LOOK

Dress nice. Use fluent hand gestures that are not attacking in any way.

—Advice to child molesters from a notorious pedophile

"I HAD A feeling that something wasn't right," twelve-year-old Mickenzie Smith said. "He was too friendly" (Smith 2005). "He" was Damon Victor Crist, twenty-two, the man who, on July 26, 2005, stopped his silver four-door pickup and approached Mickenzie and her brother Kaidan, nine, as they fed horses along a dirt road near their home in West Haven, Utah. The too-friendly stranger talked about ways to properly feed the animals, and asked for help in finding his supposedly "lost dog."

If the unfamiliar man seemed not quite right, he also seemed deceptive. When Mickenzie asked to see a photo of his dog, Crist said he thought he had one but could not produce it. He said his cell phone had died, but Mickenzie heard a mobile phone ringing in his truck. Her suspicions grew that this "friend" indeed was a friend in need of more than small talk.

A friend is someone you know, like, and trust. For Mickenzie, the danger sign was the man's premature friendliness. His physical approach was simply too forward, too soon—uninvited, unwelcome, and unwanted. Then, when he wouldn't leave, and physically blocked her path, Mickenzie's intuitions were confirmed. The friendly stranger was in fact a fiend.

As Mickenzie and Kaidan hopped on their bikes to ride away from the stranger, he blocked them, then grabbed Mickenzie and threw her into his Ford pickup. She fought back—kicked, gouged, screamed, and hit him on his head, arms, and shoulders—and prevailed. After driving less than a hundred yards, the man stopped and yelled for her to get out.

Years ago, psychologist Edward Thorndike observed that our aversion to the intrusions of strangers is innate (Thorndike 1940). Mickenzie had experienced a natural feeling of what psychologists today call "stranger anxiety"—an instinctive fear of unknown people—and trusted her instincts. First she tried to flee, and when she was trapped, she fought back. Police use Mickenzie's abduction as a textbook case of what to do when cornered: fight.

On August 1, 2005, the too-friendly stranger, multiple felon Damon Crist, was charged with child kidnapping for the attempted abduction of Mickenzie Smith. On February 16, 2006, he was sentenced to ten years to life in prison. In the predatory world of child sex abusers, Crist's case testifies to the classic parental rule: "Danger, danger—don't talk to strangers."

Yet, the typical sexual predator, an adult male between the ages of eighteen and sixty, is a man who knows his victim before the molestation takes place. He may be a family friend or an actual family member. Most often, molesters are acquaintances, trusted uncles, parents' business partners, neighbors down the street. They may be coaches, teachers, or "friends" met on the Internet. In some cases, they are local parish priests.

PREDATORY BODY LANGUAGE

Sexual predators are the most underhanded of all criminal offenders. Certainly they are the most cunning in body language, both in controlling their own signals and in reading those of others. In physical appearance, predators may be attractive, unattractive, or average-looking men. However, it's not what their faces or bodies look like that matters. Rather, it's how they behave. When you know what to look for, behavioral warning signs are easy to identify and decode. Reading a predator's crime signals enables you to stop sexual abuse before it begins.

To target his victims, a pedophile watches for nonverbal clues of vulnerability. He may test by probing with his hands. Does a child accept or pull away from a seemingly casual touch to the forearm, neck, or shoulder? Simultaneously, to cover his evil intentions, the predator gives off visible signals of honesty, decency, and virtue. He may wear the uniform of someone trustworthy, such as a Boy Scout leader, a policeman, or a priest. Dressed as a "moral leader," the wolf in sheep's clothing looks for signs of least resistance before leading a child astray.

> To target his victims, a pedophile watches for nonverbal clues of vulnerability.

We learned a lot about predatory behavior from entertainer Michael Jackson's 2005 child abuse trial in California. Though Jackson was not convicted of sexual molestation, his case was a tutorial in child harm. From expert witnesses, we learned that pedophiles establish rapport with victims with gifts, favors, and displays of personal charm. We learned how predators simultaneously dupe parents with conspicuous good deeds on behalf of their children.

We learned, in short, just how skilled these victimizers can be at using persuasive gestures, convincing facial expressions, and obliging voice tones to gain trust initially, and subsequently to cover their tracks. In this chapter, we will explore the nonverbal side of sexually abusive behavior to learn what its signals look, sound, and feel like.

You will note that in many cases, the demeanor of sex abusers resembles that of courting couples. But unlike a normal courtship, the predatory version quickly becomes secretive, demanding, coercive, and ugly. Caught in a predator's self-centered web, we will see, young victims respond with readable signs of depression, anxiety, and fear.

PREEMPTIVE TOUCHING

Like normal courting adults, child sex abusers move through a series of predictable steps. Psychologist Leigh Baker of the Trauma Treatment Center of Colorado has identified five stages in the sexual predator's progression to abuse: (1) detection, (2) approach, (3) subjugation, (4) grooming, and (5) abuse (Baker 2002). Knowing what to look for will help you see warning signs in each of the five stages.

In the detection stage, a predator prospects for new victims. As someone entrusted with responsibility for children, he carefully watches their demeanor in activity sessions or play groups to learn who is confident and who is more compliantly submissive. He may detect submissiveness in such nonverbal signs as pouting, whining, diffident shoulder shrugs, and downcast eyes. The submissive child is more likely than a self-assured youngster to listen to "parental" suggestions and follow the predator's lead.

One of the clearest warning signs in this stage is "preemptive tactile contact." In a business sense, "preemptive" refers to making prior claims on a property. In pedophilia, preemptive touching makes nonverbal claims on a child. The abuser reaches out an exploratory hand to test for physical reaction before launching his attack. While we all at times touch small children to show our affection, the abuser's touch is neither affectionate nor innocent. Rather, it is given in the guise of friendly affection to test the child's response. To a pedophile, touching is only a test.

In full view of guests at the neighborhood barbecue, a predator may use his fingers as tactile antennae to gauge a child's receptiveness to hands-on contact. Clamping sensitive pads of proprietary fingertips on the back of your son's or daughter's neck, the offender takes a reading. Should he feel shoulders lift, he'll read the involuntary shrug as a promising sign of acquiescence.

Ever since Charles Darwin's 1872 classic, *The Expression of the Emotions in Man and Animals*, the shoulder shrug has been recognized as a universal gesture of helplessness and uncertainty. In the brief shrug of submissiveness, your son or daughter unwittingly accepts the abuser's preemptive touch with a sign of vulnerability.

If your child's neck tenses, shoulders square, and body twists away instead, the pedophile will likely shift his focus and pursue a less avoidant victim at the barbecue. Seeing a man preemptively touching young children—with hands lingering longer than two or three seconds to take their reading—should make you suspicious. What looks like a minor detail of behavior could be a major cue. You may have witnessed the first telltale sign in a sequence leading down the predatory pathway.

"AIMING" THE UPPER BODY

In Leigh Baker's second stage, approach, the predator moves physically close to befriend his potential victim. He asks about the child's home life and looks again for subtle facial cues—grimaces, eyebrow raises, lip pouts—to gauge how the child feels about parents, siblings, friends, and life in general. Sadness, jealousy, misery, and problems, especially with mothers and fathers, are all exploitable. Detecting a void, the abuser stands in as an emotional replacement.

One warning sign I've observed in this stage is a powerful orientation or "aiming" of the upper body. In the postural aim, a man's face and shoulders square up with, address, and directly align with those of the child. The abuser leans close and locks onto the child's eyes to dominate with focused attention. Like a deer caught in headlights, the victim is momentarily stunned by the adult's sheer physical presence.

To children, a grown-up's bigger size, deeper voice, more commanding face, and superior communication skills lend him a natural advantage. Through the gullible eyes of a vulnerable child, adults look trustworthy, authoritative, and parental. When you see a man "aim" his body and lock onto a child, be suspicious. With so many children around, why does he orient to only one? At close quarters, his behavior is simply too intimate, exclusive, and intense for comfort.

Though not the youngster's parent, while crouched and huddled with the child the abuser appears quasi-parental. He has stepped in to substitute for the true parent. The redirection of a child's feelings for the real parent may be unconsciously triggered by another adult's matching gestures, familiar facial features, and similar tones of voice.

In psychology this is known as "transference," a phenomenon to which children are highly susceptible. Almost any adult emits some nonverbal signs that resemble those of a nurturing father, mother, or grandparent. Predators will rely on transference to garner your child's trust. Thus, when you see quasi-parental signals, beware.

SIGNS OF SUBJUGATION AND GROOMING

Success in stage two leads to stage three, subjugation. Now the predator moves into a clearer dominance mode to exert control. He positions his body closer still, stares into the child's eyes, and hypnotically fills the victim with his presence. Tone of voice, still intimate and friendly, at times turns edgy, insistent, and sharp. Dominance is tested.

At this stage, observant parents will see danger signs as the predator spends more and more time with and dotes on his victim. Again, the offender's focus appears too intense, too close for comfort. The threat level swiftly escalates as the abuser builds a "special relationship" with the victim that excludes all others. Seeing repeated invasions of a child's personal space, parents need to take charge. If you are a parent, you should act now. Step in and take control.

Should a boy or girl become trapped in a predator's web, the abuser will escalate by launching stage four, grooming. Now is the time, Baker explains, for giving expensive gifts and granting extraordinary favors as the child is groomed for the final stage, abuse. The predator will begin to test physical boundaries and reactions to affectionate touching. Since they happen in private, you may not see these intimate behaviors, and to keep you from learning about them the offender will swear the child to secrecy.

Psychologically, sharing an adult's special secret will help bond the child and predator into an exclusive pair. Sharing also deters a youngster from reporting the sexual abuse that is to come. If you suspect that your son or daughter is being groomed for abuse, ask questions about the man he or she is seeing. Has this person ever kissed, tickled, or wrestled with your child? If the answer is yes, remain calm with your youngster, but confront the adult. Let him know in the clearest of terms that touching is taboo, and that spending time alone together is henceforth forbidden.

ABUSIVE TICKLING

Learning that your child has been tickled by a man should raise major concerns. In *Love Signals,* I wrote that tickling is a widespread behavior in the fourth or touch phase of courtship (Givens 2005). As a playful cue, tickling is often seen in child-child, parent-child, and courting-adult pairs. The harmless-seeming, "unserious" quality of tickling has made it an ideal form of touch communication in courtship.

Heavy tickling, called "gargalesis," in which the skin of the ribs or waist is indented by another's poking fingertips, usually produces the laugh response. Tickling the neck, armpits, and sides of the abdomen may also arouse sexual feelings as it stimulates nonspecific erogenous areas of skin.

For a glimpse of tickling's abusive side, consider the case of former Catholic priest Patrick G. O'Donnell. In his July 7 and August 30, 2004, sworn depositions in Seattle, Washington, O'Donnell admitted that he had sexually molested boys on Boy Scout trips, on church property, and at other locations in Washington State and Idaho (De Leon 2004).

As per sworn statements of his adult accusers, the touches they received from O'Donnell as teenagers started with massage, playful wrestling, or tickling. In his own deposition, the ex-priest described one such tickling match that took place in Spokane: "We got down under the pants to—either to the genitals or almost to the genitals" (De Leon 2004).

Innocent tickling may be just that: innocent. But for child sex abusers, tickling is a certain danger sign.

SIGNS OF SEXUAL ABUSE

In the final stage, abuse, the predator physically attacks his victim. In her book *Protecting Your Children from Sexual Predators*, Baker cites the case of "Mr. Bob" and five-year-old Jensen, whom he had earlier approached, subjugated, and groomed. Sitting in his car on a cold spring day, Mr. Bob enacted every parent's nightmare. He invited Jensen closer so they both could keep warm. Sitting the little boy down on his lap, the man proceeded to touch Jensen inappropriately. Though not his real father, Mr. Bob told Jensen that this was a "normal" way for fathers to teach their little boys about sex. After the molestation, he swore Jensen to secrecy, lest the parents send Mr. Bob away forever and put little Jensen in a foster home (Baker 2002, 53).

The predator's fear tactics worked. He continued abusing Jensen for another three months. During that time, the boy's mother began to notice nonverbal signs of abuse: clinging, needy behavior, isolating himself in his room, bed-wetting, wetting his pants in school, and thumb sucking. When she asked if anyone had touched him, he was unable to speak. Finally, after his mother reassured Jensen that she loved him and would never send him away, he told her the truth.

It is a tribute to the boy's mother that she finally noticed, read, and accurately decoded the crime signals, freeing her son from his monstrous ordeal. Had she read them earlier in the five-stage progression to abuse, Jensen and his family could have avoided a great deal of emotional pain.

Recognizing behavioral signs that precede sex abuse will help you guard against predators who would target your children. Be suspicious of any adult who finagles a way to spend time alone with your child through babysitting, travel to sports events, or trips to the shopping mall. Jensen was molested on trips away from his parents, in the privacy of Mr. Bob's car. When confronting any predator face-to-face, expect nonverbal deception. Again, abusers are cunning in body language and unusually able to control their nonverbal responses.

"If a sex offender is breathing who doesn't know to keep good eye contact when he's lying," psychologist Anna Salter writes, "I haven't met him yet." As a man who had raped dozens of children confided to her, "The manner that I use when I was trying to convince somebody—even though I knew I was lying— I'd look them in the eye, but I wouldn't stare at them. Staring makes people uncomfortable and that tends to turn them away, so I wouldn't stare at them. But look at them in a manner that, you know, 'look at this innocent face. How can you believe that I would do something like that?'" (Salter 2003, 39).

The best way to stop child sex abuse is to step in before it begins. Heed the nonverbal signs of a predator's approach, subjugation, and grooming phases. If possible, stop him in the approach stage before he subdues, grooms, and ultimately abuses.

Be extremely suspicious of any man who surrounds himself with children and gives special favors to a few. In 2004, a suspected sexual predator was identified by the special favors he showed at Holy Cross Lutheran Church in Spokane. A mother became concerned when she noticed her teenage daughter's youth pastor "paying attention to just the females in the youth group" (Clouse 2005). She notified church officials, who mandated psychological counseling for the thirty-one-year-old man. Shortly after, unbeknownst to the mother, the suspect allegedly contacted her daughter on the Internet and persuaded the teenage girl to expose her body on the family's Web cam.

After an investigation, police arrested pastor James Ritter charging him with first-degree sexual misconduct with a minor, sexual exploitation of a minor, and communication with a minor for immoral purposes. Had the teen's mom not noticed him giving special favors to girls, his predation would have continued. What looked like a relatively minor detail of behavior, favoritism, turned out to be a telling cue.

CASE STUDIES: A TALE OF TWO PRIESTS

The overwhelming majority of people who sexually abuse children are men. Among the most trustworthy of men, one might assume, are Catholic priests. But the thousands of lawsuits in the United States against allegedly abusive priests suggest otherwise. Just what kinds of signals do priests send to lure their victims? For answers, let's see how two notoriously abusive priests displayed visual, tactile, auditory—even chemical—signs when they trolled for victims.

Clergy Case I

An admitted sexual predator, former Catholic priest Patrick G. O'Donnell of Washington State sent tactile and visual signals. In touching, he massaged, wrestled with, and tickled his victims. Visually, O'Donnell used another common sex-offender ploy: he exhibited his own body as bait. Had parents known O'Donnell was an exhibitionist, they might have kept their sons from going on unsupervised trips with him.

Exhibitionism is the psychological need to show one's naked body, especially genitalia, to other people. It can be blatant, like that of the thirty-two-year-old Spokane man who in October 2005 was cited for indecent exposure while walking around naked in front of a large cardboard box with "Sex Wanted" written on its side. Or it can be subtle, like that of Father O'Donnell.

From 1976 to 1978, O'Donnell played racquetball with young boys at Seattle University, and would shower with them afterward. "That was part of the deal with him," recalls Jim Biteman, now a middle-aged man, who was an eighth-grader at the time (Shapiro 2002). Biteman went on to tell how O'Donnell would go nude on his cabin cruiser and showily swing himself into the lake as boys onboard watched.

If O'Donnell was something of an exhibitionist, he was also a voyeur. A voyeur is someone who obtains sexual gratification from seeing the naked bodies of others. According to his church, O'Donnell took part in a questionable sponge-bath incident with boys in the junior high school adjoining his Spokane parish (Shapiro 2002). On other occasions, according to Biteman, O'Donnell would encourage boys to go for nude swims off his boat in Seattle's Lake Washington. "He would sit in the back of the boat," Biteman recalled, "and encourage us to jump in and get out, jump in and get out" (Shapiro 2002).

The sight of the priest's naked body and the delight he showed watching boys' naked bodies were clear warning signs that sexual abuse would take place. The predator's body language left little doubt as to what he would, could, and finally did do. In addition, ominous signals were evident in O'Donnell's proxemic behavior. Anthropologist Edward Hall identified an "intimate" zone in which lovers and family members interact in close physical proximity, zero to eighteen inches away. O'Donnell planned each of his sporting, boating, camping, Boy Scout, and Catholic Youth Ministry activities with a single goal in mind: to attain intimate physical closeness with his victims. To parents, his pattern of surrounding himself with young boys should have been a clear danger sign.

Clergy Case II

Sexual predator Michael Edwin Wempe, a retired priest from the Roman Catholic Archdiocese of Los Angeles, displayed tactile, auditory, and chemical signs with the thirteen boys he seduced and molested in the 1970s and 1980s.

Known for his flamboyant long hair, motorcycle, and hipster ways, Wempe preyed on boys from needy families by giving gifts and invitations to fancy dinners. He took them on adventures shooting, camping, water skiing, and deep-sea fishing, and rode with them on his motorcycle. There was always the motorcycle. Its speed, acceleration, and engine roar excited and filled the senses of his young passengers.

After strategically cultivating parental trust, Father Michael would take his victims for motorcycle rides and then boldly reach into their pants. "My hands are cold," he told one of the boys (Garrison and Guccione 2006a). Afterward, he violated victims in his bed at the rectory, in camp, or wherever they slept.

One of the victims, a former altar boy who testified as a forty-year-old man that he'd endured five years of the priest's abuse, said Wempe took him snow skiing and to golf tournaments, and gave him a ride to San Simeon's Hearst Castle on his motorcycle (Garrison and Guccione 2006a).

Wempe used a similar pattern of gifting, befriending, attention giving, and special treatment with each of his victims. A key ingredient in the priest's seduction was adrenaline. He took boys on thrilling, adrenaline-charged trips down the highway aboard his motorcycle. According to Los Angeles County deputy district attorney Todd Hicks, "he was well-practiced. He followed this pattern religiously" (Garrison and Guccione 2006a).

The chemical adrenaline ($C_9H_{13}NO_3$) heightens sexual attraction. Priests and boys stand a better chance of bonding when they share an emotionally exciting moment together.

For the child, arousal due to excitement on the highway was mistaken for arousal due to sexual attraction. Since chemically induced feelings of exhilaration and arousal are "nonspecific," they are easily confused. Arousal from cycle riding together—triggering release of adrenaline into the bloodstream—feels like arousal from infatuation. In both, adrenal hormones increase heart rate, blood pressure, blood sugar, and metabolism to fuel the thrill.

Michael Wempe would open with adrenaline and follow up with touch. Touching began on the road and continued after the trips. A twenty-six-year-old man weepingly testified that as a boy, "he thought it was normal that the priest touched his genitals. 'It was Father Mike. It was really difficult to think that anything he did could be wrong'" (Garrison and Guccione 2006b). It was wrong, of course, and on February 22, 2006, Michael Edwin Wempe, sixty-six, was convicted of child molestation in Los Angeles County Superior Court.

Like all sexual predators, priests employ multimodal signals—visual, tactile, auditory, and excitatory—to entice their victims. Know both what the signs are and what they say. To safeguard your child, understand what people in positions of authority do rather than what they themselves say. As always, actions speak louder than words. Since the crime signals your child sees are often hidden from you, don't be afraid to ask the *t* question: "Does your new friend ever touch you?" As you listen, watch your youngster's hands, shoulders, lips, and eyes for the deception cues we explored in chapter 2. Seen in the context of a probing question about being touched, they show that you both may now have a problem.

PREDATORY ROMANCES

Along with pretend "parents" and abusive priests, boyfriends can be dangerous sexual predators. In the United States, a third of all girls between the ages of ten and eighteen report having been assaulted by their boyfriends. But like others in this subterranean zone of the criminal world, boyfriends give off readable danger signs before and after their crimes. Parents of teenage girls need to read them and take heed.

Beware the romantic grand gesture, the overdone display of affection proffered from a distance. Rather than address her personally, face-to-face, the hopeful suitor launches an inappropriately grandiose message from afar. Grand gestures are imaginative but hardly infallible. On January 4, 2006, Spokane County resident Terra Florian testified that Thomas Crook, forty-two, sent flowers and a pizza to her workplace in a limousine (Craig 2006a). After refusing the man's chauffeured gifts, Florian began to receive harassing phone calls, death threats, and misdirected visits from pizza drivers, taxicabs, and plumbers. On January 9, 2006, Mr. Crook was found guilty in superior court of felony stalking and harassment (Craig 2006b).

Body-language "before" signs are visible in boyfriends who are overly charming, overly macho, and behave too politely (at first) with their girlfriends' parents. Offending boyfriends give too many gifts, display intense possessiveness, and exhibit raging outbursts of jealousy. They belittle, manipulate, and flagrantly dominate their girlfriends. A predatory boyfriend will strive to remake his steady's physical appearance; to dictate her clothing, hairstyle, and makeup; and to isolate her from friends and family. On the verbal side, after insulting or physically attacking he will say, "I love you."

A predatory boyfriend makes unannounced home visits and frequent phone calls in which he raises his voice, cries, or threatens. Actual assault comes next. He may shove, slap, hit, punch, bite, kick, or choke his girlfriend, as well as twist her arm, pull her hair, wrestle her to the floor, throw her against a wall, or push her from his car. He breaks and enters, steals, stalks, curses, smashes objects, punches walls and doors, glares, takes her money, blackmails, and threatens to commit suicide if she leaves.

As if these behaviors were not enough, he displays weapons, aggressively flirts with other girls in her presence, and frequently breaks up and then remorsefully returns, bearing gifts (often flowers).

APOLOGY ROSES

"**A**nd of course there are the roses. They appear and reappear in many of the girls' stories. They have come to represent a potent symbol of apology for abuse." So writes Vicki Crompton in her book *Saving Beauty from the Beast* (Crompton and Kessner 2003, 20). Vicki Crompton's teenage daughter, Jenny, was stabbed to death in her home by boyfriend Mark Smith on September 26, 1986. Before her death, Mark often gave Jenny roses as he apologized for his abusive outbreaks.

If body-language "before" signs are bad, "after" signs are worse. Nonverbal signals include visible red marks on the girlfriend's skin, choke marks on her neck, a swollen face, blue bruises, black eyes, a smashed nose, broken bones, chipped teeth, and cigarette burns. Psychologically, sharing secrets about his violent acts helps them bond together—like child abuser and abused child—as an exclusive pair. You will see significant changes in the young woman's demeanor and bearing. There will be chronic weeping, fewer outside activities, less contact with friends.

Sexually, there may be repeated coercion, aggression, servitude, and rape. Signs of post-traumatic stress disorder (PTSD) may appear. PTSD was first detected in war veterans who experienced heavy combat. Now, the American Psychiatric Association reports it in civilians, especially in females, usually within three months of a boyfriend-induced trauma. There are problems sleeping, unusual risk-taking behaviors, and recurrent nightmares and visual flashbacks, along with emotional detachment, depression, substance abuse, and avoidance of family, friends, and places where the abuse took place. In body language, one of the more visible signs to watch for is an exaggerated startle reflex.

EXAGGERATED STARTLE CUES

The startle reflex is a sudden, involuntary movement made in response to a touch, unexpected motion, or loud noise. It includes a set of automatic protective movements designed to withdraw the body and its parts away from perceived harm. Startle cues, which increase with anxiety and fatigue, are often seen in young people who have been sexually abused.

Eccentric twisting, plunging, blinking, and flexing spasms are visible in children with exaggerated startles. Defensive shoulder shrugs, eyeblinks, and facial grimaces, along with flexing motions of the neck, elbows, trunk, and knees, appear when children feel physically, emotionally, or socially threatened (Andermann and Andermann 1992, 498).

Sudden onset of startle behaviors in a daughter with a new boyfriend could be a warning sign—a nonverbal cry for your help.

On November 10, 1994, Vicki Crompton visited Mark Smith—the boyfriend killer of her teenage daughter, Jenny—at the Iowa State Men's Reformatory at Anamosa, where Mark is serving a life sentence without possibility of parole. As she wrote in *Saving Beauty from the Beast:* "He opens his palms as if begging me to understand: 'I [boyfriend Mark] was filled with uncontrollable rage—like a rush—I was all pumped up.' *Not on drugs—just adrenaline—the thrill of the kill, the high of 'I have the power to make you die'*" (Crompton and Kessner 2003, 240).

Vicki Crompton saw, read, and interpreted many of Mark Smith's crime signals, but was ultimately powerless to prevent her daughter's death. The signs Vicki saw showed clear and present danger, but like many abused daughters, Jenny did not share everything with her mother. Though she talked openly about having sex, Vicki said, "she kept Mark's violence a secret" (Crompton and Kessner 2003, 6).

Mark killed Jenny behind a veil of shared secrecy. Seeing possible signs of abuse, parents should ask daughters probing questions about their boyfriends. Does the boyfriend lash out in anger with his hands? Does he slap, punch, or kick? If the answer is yes, be on her side and step in.

FAMILY SIGNS OF ABUSE

Secrecy, isolation, and dominance are major themes in the behavior of all sexual predators. The sexual abuse of children, always horrific, is worse in incest. Incest is the statutory crime of sexual relations with a near relative. A father who abuses a daughter—the most highly reported case of incest—so undermines trust that victims become suicidal.

In father-daughter abuse, the nonverbal cue that stands out most, ironically, is secrecy. A secret is about keeping something hidden, secluded, or concealed from view. While all predators are secretive, family predators are the most secretive of all. They may conceal their misdeeds by secluding the entire family. Doors are kept locked, curtains kept closed, and children kept inside.

As a social worker in Seattle, my wife, Doreen, did home visits on behalf of children throughout the city. When she entered darkly curtained, secretive homes, she knew the families had something to hide. On occasion the something was incest or family rape. In a case she described as being "just creepy," Doreen visited the family of an abusive father named "Squiggy," thirty-five, who smiled and flirted with her but treated his wife neglectfully, "like wallpaper." Heavy, dark curtains covered the front windows, which were overgrown with moist green Seattle moss.

Squiggy locked the front door each time Doreen came inside to work with his two baby girls. The home was dark, damp, and cold, without heat, telephone, or TV. Squiggy took snapshots of my wife, and recorded her voice on tape. Oddly, he weighed his girls before and after they ate and after he'd changed their diapers. Doreen watched a compulsive, controlling father who dominated his family in the most minute aspects of their daily lives. She reported feeling unsafe in the home, and suspected the girls were being sexually abused. She was not surprised to learn, at her final home visit, that Squiggy was no longer there. He had been jailed for raping his wife's mother, who lived with the family in their enshrouded south Seattle home. Incarceration has brought Squiggy's secretive family life to an end.

Secrecy has its own behavioral signs. To those who recognize them—a thick blanket nailed over a window, a porch light habitually off, a neighbor who never looks your way and has children who never come out—such clues clearly merit attention. Secretive signals should bring close notice. What might be going on in the cloistered household? Prevented from escaping, damning information stays inside. Child incest within could stay concealed for years. When you see signs of familial secrecy, monitor the home as you would your neighbor's in a routine block watch. On behalf of the children, report unusual yelling, crying, or screaming to police.

To explore the nonverbal signs of incest, let's look at a shocking case that took place in Salisbury, Massachusetts, over a six-year period that finally ended in 2001. Visible signals of awful crimes—beatings and daily rapes by a father of his three daughters, sometimes in full view of other family members—were abundant (Anonymous 2005a). Abundant, that is, inside the home. Outside the home they were shrouded. The signals were hidden behind heavily curtained windows and guarded by an eight-foot fence. What happened inside the compound stayed inside.

Patrick McMullen held his wife, Christine, and their six children as virtual prisoners. The kids rarely left home, could not ride bikes in the front yard, and were not permitted to attend school or even to seek a doctor's care. So complete was their isolation that the children had no birth certificates, no school transcripts, and no medical records. Like the father's concealed crime signals, the family itself seemed not to exist.

Within this hermetically hidden dwelling, McMullen's crimes went on unchecked. His oldest daughter testified that her father regularly raped her for six years between 1995 and 2001. In some instances, he raped her in front of siblings. When one of the daughters was asked at what point the incest had begun, she replied that she just grew up with it.

On February 18, 2005, Patrick McMullen, forty-one, was convicted of criminal child rape and sentenced to forty years in prison. When he walked into the courtroom that day to hear the verdict, he glared at his family; when the verdict was read, he showed no visible reaction and gave no body-language cues of remorse.

Prosecutor Kathe Tuttman called McMullens' case the "most horrific" she'd ever worked on. The essential problem was the father's skill in hiding his family from public view. Yet luckily, like most predators, he'd left a crack in the compound through which crime signals finally showed. For reasons unknown, he let his wife join the Mormon Church.

Breaking the vow of silence her husband imposed, Christine McMullen told church members about his chronic violence and incest. Later, on a day when her husband was out of the home, she telephoned church members at her Latter-Day Saint stake in Exeter, New Hampshire. They came immediately to rescue Christine and her family. The father's incestuous days were over at last.

Like an astronomical black hole, McMullen's densely shrouded compound kept light from escaping. Neighbors didn't know a family even lived in that tiny slice of Salisbury. The church learned of incest there only after Christine resolutely broke through her husband's secretive wall. With brave initiative, even a black hole may be detected. Had crime signals not escaped, the McMullen home may have become a killing zone.

PREDATORY MURDER SIGNS

Let's step a rung lower now, into the very basement of the predator's subterranean world. When criminals on this bottom level sexually abuse, they kill their victims. Unlike the predators we've seen so far, these men spend little time wooing, courting, or grooming. You will not see testing with the hands, playful tickling, gift exchanges, or road trips to Hearst Castle.

Serial sexual murderers attack total strangers with little warning. They are what I call "ambush killers." In chapter 4, we saw how mass murderer Charles Whitman ambushed fourteen people from his sniper's post atop the University of Texas Tower. While Whitman gave off clearly readable crime signals before the shootings, the only signs available to victims on the ground were stinging bullets.

Like Charles Whitman, ambush killers kill before their victims have a chance to respond. In October 2002, ten men and women were randomly killed by ambush at gas stations, retail stores, and parking lots in Virginia, Maryland, and Washington, D.C. Several were shot while pumping gas. On October 14, Linda Franklin, forty-seven, an FBI intelligence analyst, was shot dead at a Home Depot in Fairfax County, Virginia. Like other victims of the Beltway Snipers, she never knew what hit her.

Perpetrators John A. Muhammad and Lee B. Malvo used a long-distance Bushmaster XM-15 semiautomatic .223 caliber rifle for their ambush murders. They fired from within the closed trunk of a former police car, a dark blue 1990 Chevrolet Caprice, through a hole cut in the vehicle's rear end. Victims had no clue they were under attack until they felt bullets piercing their flesh.

The sexual predators you are about to meet are also ambush killers. They, too, killed with little or no warning. But unlike Whitman, Muhammad, and Malvo, who murdered randomly from a distance, sexual murderers attack in close proximity, within confined quarters of a personal killing zone established inside a vehicle, dormitory, or bedroom. Instead of high-powered rifles, they use hatchets, knives, pistols, or their own bare hands. Their homicides are up close and personal, committed within the proxemic boundaries of Edward Hall's "intimate zone," zero to eighteen inches apart.

To learn more about the predatory behavior of sexual murderers, let's consider three infamous predators from Washington State: Theodore Bundy, Robert Yates, and Gary Ridgway (the "Green River Killer"). What body language did these serial predators use to lure dozens of young women to their deaths?

Though each was a serial killer, none of the men physically chased their victims, ran them down on foot, broke into their homes, or wrestled them to the ground. On the contrary, Ted Bundy used visibly submissive behavior. He politely asked for help and feigned physical injury with crutches, counterfeit casts, and a fake limp. Yates and Ridgway used a businesslike demeanor to bargain for sex acts with cash. If, with his vulnerable come-on, Bundy seemed obsequious, Yates and Ridgway seemed like "regular guys."

When victims were securely confined inside the men's vehicles, the three predators behaved alike. They sprang from needy, gentlemanly, or regular-guy disguises to kill with a crowbar, shoot with a pistol, or strangle with bare hands. Each man abruptly shifted from his "harmless" persona into lethal ambush mode. Each attacked suddenly from behind a front of seemingly benign demeanor.

To abduct his victims, Ted Bundy would approach unacquainted women to ask for assistance. Bundy was handsome, well educated, and articulate, and his requests must have seemed benign at the time. Nonverbally, he used a diffident, submissive approach to seem harmless and keep victims from avoiding him or running away. To enlist sympathy, Bundy used body language of the handicapped, disabled, and walking wounded. He stepped with a limp, or used crutches and wore a plaster cast.

On November 8, 1974, Ted Bundy approached a young woman at a high school auditorium in Utah and asked for her assistance in identifying a car. She refused, and later said something had seemed odd or scary about the man (Bell 2006). Perhaps it boiled down to his persistence. He'd physically approached her twice, then hung around in back of the auditorium as if waiting to approach her a third time. Unlike a truly vulnerable man, a predatory man feigns submissiveness to appear vulnerable. But note a key difference in nonverbal behavior. The harmless-seeming predator will aggressively pursue his targeted victim, repeatedly approach, and persistently step forward into her path. Biologists would see Bundy's persistence as an alternative form of aggression. In the wild kingdom, it's often the case that persistent animals, not the strongest or most powerful, win the battle.

Bundy's favorite killing zone was the cramped interior of his Volkswagen Bug. When an unsuspecting woman stepped into his meek-looking Beetle, Ted would drive away and then kill her with blows to her head with a tire iron or hatchet, or by strangulation. The horrors didn't stop there. Once she was dead, he might have sex with the cadaver and keep the head as a trophy. On January 24, 1989, after confessing to the murders of twenty-three young women across the United States between 1974 and 1978, Theodore Bundy, forty-two, was put to death for his crimes in Florida's electric chair.

Like Bundy, Robert Yates Jr. kept trophies. Yates buried one of his female victims beneath his—and his wife's—bedroom on Spokane's South Hill. Gary Ridgway, too, kept trophy cadavers. He hid them in wooded areas near Seattle's Green River, and periodically drove by to view them and reminisce. Trophy taking plays into the need to sequester victims in private kill zones beforehand. Sequestering bodies makes it easier for predators to claim them as private property after the murders.

At the trial of Robert Lee Yates Jr., prostitutes testified that Yates behaved like a gentleman, paid up front, used a condom, and did not assault them. In Christine Smith's case, however, he attacked. She was the only woman to escape from one of Yates's attacks. On August 1, 1998, Smith got into Yates's black Ford van to transact a sex-for-fee deal. When Smith and Yates agreed to $40 for oral sex, he handed her the payment in cash. Smith told the jury that Yates just "looked like a normal, everyday man."

In the confines of Yates's killing zone—the inner sanctum of his black Ford van—Christine was suddenly struck in the back of the head, causing her to feel a spinning sensation and experience blurred vision. Perhaps due to intoxication or drug use, she didn't hear the sound of a gun, but bullet fragments were later found in her skull. After the shooting, which Smith managed to survive, Yates asked her to give him all of her money. In the ensuing confusion, she managed to escape from his van.

At their 2002 reunion in court, body language revealed what words did not. "From his chair," Bill Morlin wrote in the Spokane (Wash.) *Spokesman-Review*, "Yates made eye contact with the witness [Christine Smith], but continued his emotionless gaze, occasionally looking downward. She smiled back, pursing her lips" (Morlin 2002). Emotionless eyes revealed a guilty man unable to dispute the witness's claims. His downward gaze revealed psychic abdication. Meanwhile, Christine's pursed-lipped smile seemed to say, "I win, little man."

After killing his victims, Yates would have sex with some, then dump their bodies near where he'd found them. Yates finally confessed to committing fifteen murders. Twelve were female prostitutes murdered in Spokane from 1996 to 1998. On September 19, 2002, Yates, fifty, was found guilty in Tacoma, Washington, of aggravated first-degree murder for killing two young Tacoma women. On October 3, 2002, Yates received the death sentence for his crimes. As he heard the sentence, he meekly bowed his head.

On November 5, 2003, Gary Leon Ridgway, fifty-four, confessed to the murders of forty-eight women from 1982 to 1998, mostly prostitutes. Agreeing to provide information to authorities about his victims, he was sentenced on December 18, 2003, to life in prison without parole.

Like Yates, Ridgway propositioned young women for sex in return for cash. Prostitutes would enter his truck of their own volition. During or soon after sex, Ridgway would strangle them in his home or in the dense stands of trees and blackberries south of Seattle near the Green River. Some bodies were thrown into the river, while others were put in the woods so he could drive by and recall his killings.

> **Choking was what I did, and I was pretty good at it.**
> —Gary Ridgway (who considered choking "more personal and more rewarding than to shoot her")

Within personally demarcated killing zones, predatory murderers do lethal harm by ambushing victims in close proximity from behind false fronts of benign demeanor. Nonverbally, they seem like ordinary men until you are physically alone with them inside a confined, private, circumscribed space. Once inside, killing begins. Being inside almost any place together—a van, a kitchen, a dorm room—establishes the psychological confinement the murderer needs to set up his kill zone. Being alone with you inside empowers him to take your life.

This kind of predator feels physically strong inside his zone. Outside its boundaries, he feels weak. He is not aggressive enough to break down your door or smash through a window to get you. Breaking and entering is not his style. He does not become aggressive until his proxemic surroundings seem right. Like a spider, he won't physically chase you, but trapped in his web you become as helpless as a fly. Being alone with you inside puts him in control.

To protect yourself and your family from sex abusers, be alert to their crime signals and stay off their predatory pathways. Here are some signals to be especially wary of:

- Unwarranted gifts, favors, and displays of personal charm
- Uninvited, unwelcome, unwanted physical approaches
- Preemptive touching with the hands
- Adult-child touching, playful wrestling, tickling
- Suspicious bruises, chipped teeth, cigarette burns
- An exaggerated startle reflex

As terrible as sexual predators are, some offenders—as measured by the sheer destructive quality of their deeds—are even worse. In the next chapter, we study the body language of religious and fanatical terrorists.

7

TERROR INTERRUPTED

She noticed that Ressam was acting strangely, and followed her hunch.

—A U.S. terrorist hunter's comment
on a U.S. Customs officer in Washington State

"HE GAVE ME THE CREEPS"

"When the subject looked at me, I felt a bone chilling cold effect," customs inspector Jose Melendez-Perez told the U.S. 9/11 Commission. "The bottom line is, he gave me the creeps" (Melendez-Perez 2004).

The suspicious man in question was Saudi national Mohamed al-Kahtani, who on August 4, 2001, arrived at Florida's Orlando International Airport (MCO) aboard a Virgin Atlantic Airways flight from London. Jose Melendez-Perez, a U.S. immigration inspector at MCO, was assigned to interview al-Kahtani, who had an authentic Saudi passport and a valid U.S. visa.

Inspector Melendez-Perez's first impression was of a well-groomed, very muscular young man with short hair and a trimmed mustache. Dressed in black shirt, black trousers, and black shoes, Mohamed al-Kahtani projected a militant bearing. "Upon establishing eye contact," Melendez-Perez reported, "he exhibited body language and facial gestures that appeared arrogant. In fact, when I first called his name in the secondary room and matched him with papers, he had a deep staring look" (Melendez-Perez 2004).

An experienced immigration inspector, Jose Melendez-Perez had also been trained in deciphering body language. His first question to Mohamed, posed through an interpreter, was to ask why he'd traveled without a return airline ticket. According to Jose, "The subject became visibly upset and in an arrogant and threatening manner, which included pointing his finger at my face, stated that he did not know where he was going when he departed the United States" (Melendez-Perez 2004). Based on this answer, Jose considered the suspect a "hit man," which is to say, an agent on a mission who was not told beforehand where to go. This way, in case of capture, he would have no information or leads to give police.

Mohamed al-Kahtani told Melendez-Perez he was going to stay in a hotel. Yet he had no credit cards, no hotel reservations, and just $2,800 in cash. "Just," because the return flight home would cost $2,200. He told Melendez-Perez he planned to stay in the U.S. for six days, and that he'd been instructed to call someone who would arrange for someone else to pick him up. When Jose asked who the first someone was, al-Kahtani gruffly stated that it was a personal matter and none of his business. "The subject was very hostile throughout the entire interview that took approximately 1½ hours," Melendez-Perez told the commission (Melendez-Perez 2004).

Based on the Saudi visitor's confrontational body language, visible hostility, and evasiveness—he claimed to be on a "vacation tour" of the U.S., yet refused to give details about his itinerary, personal contacts, or means of support—al-Kahtani was advised that he didn't appear to be admissible to the United States. When given the opportunity to voluntarily withdraw his application, he did so, and signed an official I-275 form. On August 4, 2001, the day of his arrival, the creepy young man departed Orlando via Virgin Atlantic Airways to London, with a connecting flight to Dubai. "Before boarding the aircraft," Jose told the commission, "the subject turned to [the] other inspector and myself and said, in English, something to the effect of, 'I'll be back' " (Melendez-Perez 2004).

Investigators later learned the man Mohamed al-Kahtani was to meet in Orlando was none other than Mohammed Atta, a lead terrorist in the September 11, 2001, attacks. Atta had been waiting for al-Kahtani inside the Orlando airport. The 9/11 Commission concluded that Mohamed al-Kahtani had likely been assigned as the "twentieth hijacker," to fly on the United Airlines plane that crashed on September 11 in Pennsylvania. It crashed because passengers fought the hijackers on board, preventing them from striking one of two likely targets, the White House or the U.S. Capitol. Had Jose Melendez-Perez not noticed something evil in al-Kahtani's glaring eyes, the terrorist might have boarded the jetliner. Had he added his substantial muscle to the hijack team, it might have reached Washington, D.C., and destroyed a key national landmark.

SIGNS OF FEAR

A terrorist's crime signals send overt messages. The word "terror" means "intense, overpowering fear." A terrorist is therefore someone who uses panic, intimidation, or gratuitous violence to influence governments, religious groups, or rival factions.

Fear is a usually unpleasant visceral feeling of anxiety, apprehension, or dread. In evolutionary terms, it is a mammalian elaboration of the sympathetic nervous system's fight-or-flight response. Fear makes us feel like attacking or running away. It shows in the face, body, voice, and eyes. Among the most noticed physical signs of fear are hurried breathing, trembling hands, pale skin, cold sweat, chattering teeth, cowering, crying, rapid blinking, frozen body movements, bristling hair, violent heartbeat, rigidly tightened muscles, screaming, squirming, sweaty palms, staring with dilated pupils, audibly strained voice tones, throat clearing, tensed lips, facial self-touching, jaw drooping, and widely opened "flashbulb eyes."

Fear shows in one's face, body movements, voice, and eyes.

The last three signs of fear in the above list are seen in the clasped cheeks, open mouth, and staring eyes of *The Scream*, a painting completed in 1893 by Norwegian artist Edvard Munch. A cultural icon of humankind's rising fright level, *The Scream* could serve as terrorism's trademark.

Oddly, we can also enjoy vicarious feelings of fear, as in movies. For instance, the most-portrayed movie character of all time is Bram Stoker's Dracula. To date, over 155 representations of the evil Count Dracula have appeared on the screen (McFarlan 1990, 165).

But while fear can be thrilling as entertainment, in terrorism it's too scary for words. The Provisional Irish Republican Army shot enemies in the kneecap for revenge, and to use their victims' crippled body language as a constant reminder of terrorist threat.

In Italy, shooting in the leg—called *azzoppanento*, or "laming"—sends the same message. While dead men tell no tales, the walking wounded keep terror alive.

TERRORIZING WITH COLOR

Colors beam information about emotions, feelings, and moods. Wearing the same color suggests shared membership in a group, tribe, or gang. National states mark their identity with colorful dyes affixed to banners, crests, and flags.

Terrorists use colors to frighten. The practice is rooted in prehistory. Tribal warriors, like men of the Karo tribe in Ethiopia, wear white, brown, and orange face paint to intimidate. Tairora men of Papua New Guinea wear colorful, vertically ascending headgear to loom larger than life. Fatah's menacing flag is black, white, green, and red. Black suggests fear, white suggests cold, green signifies hate, and red shows defiance (Richmond et al. 1991). In what may be the functional equivalent of war paint, some terrorist groups include inciting colors in their names: Black September, Red Army Faction, Red Brigades, and Red Hand Defenders.

An early terrorist color was brown. Worn on the body, brown is not a tender hue. It evokes moods of sadness and dejection. Symbolically, brown suggests melancholy, atonement, and decay. In the world of terror, brown stands for fear.

In Munich, Germany, Adolf Hitler led his right-wing followers—who dressed in boots, riding pants, and brown shirts—in a failed battle to topple the German government and seize power in 1923, sixteen years before World War II. Released from prison after the attempted putsch, Hitler mobilized his Brownshirts as storm troopers. Attacking Catholics, Gypsies, Jews, and anyone who got in their path, they noisily marched through German streets carrying black flags emblazoned with white skulls and crossbones.

Dressing alike in uniforms gave Hitler's Brownshirts the look and feel of a unified team. Since black on white is one of the most visible color contrasts the human eye can see, the Brownshirts' flag brought attention to their presence on the streets and signaled their collective identity. That the flag's movement and flutter seemed lifelike to vision centers of the brain intensified the Brownshirts' terror.

Waved by death-dealing Brownshirts, pirate flags symbolized the stark terror of Hermann Goering's words. Goering, first chief of the Brownshirts, said, "I have no obligation to abide by the law; my job is simply to annihilate and exterminate" (Nash 1998).

VIGILANT OBSERVATIONS

As the threat of international terrorism grows, nonverbal communication plays a vital role in the training of government, military, and law-enforcement personnel. The ability to see danger signs in anomalous behaviors, atypical body movements, and unusual clothing is essential for public safety today.

The best observers rely on their own feelings to ask questions: "Why do those men seem nervous? Why do they make me feel nervous? Why are they walking single file instead of side by side—are they on a mission?" If you guessed that they were on a mission, your instincts might be correct. U.S. Border Patrol officers identify walking in line as a warning sign of intentions to cross a national border illegally as a team.

United Airlines does annual training to help its flight attendants watch for unusual behaviors in nervous passengers. Their years of experience allow them to spot abnormal signals— deviations from the norm. In a commercial aircraft, flight attendants monitor anxiety as a warning sign of possible deviate intentions.

From thousands of hours flying, attendants internalize an
"experiential blueprint" for what is normal.

Software has been developed to interpret nonverbal behavior captured on closed-circuit cameras. Computers can distinguish between normal and abnormal conduct. To remain in an airport elevator longer than sixty seconds would set off a security alarm. Odd behavior within the elevator, such as raising both hands together—as if to affix an explosive device overhead—would do the same. The timing of a terrorist act can be telling as well. Retired FBI special agent Joe Navarro notes that a mission may be timed to begin at the top of the hour. As the zero hour—9:00 a.m., say—nears, individual readiness to act shows prior to concerted action. Just before 9:00 a.m., bodies stand taller, motions become faster, and gestures seem tense as demeanor telegraphs heightened arousal (Navarro 2006).

A CLASSIC CASE OF NONVERBAL SURVEILLANCE

Consider the case of Ahmed Ressam, an Algerian loner who crossed into Washington State from Canada on the Port Angeles ferry on December 14, 1999. Ressam's was the last car off the ferryboat, and something in his body language told customs inspector Diana Dean to take a closer look (Anonymous 2001).

Ressam appeared nervous and sweaty. Dean gave him a declaration form and asked him to step out of his car. In the words of officers on the scene, Ressam's "hemming" (speech hesitations), "hawing" (fumbling for words), "dawdling" (taking more time than necessary), and "stalling" (using delay tactics) drew inspector Mark Johnson's attention (Johnson 2001).

Ressam got out of his car and stood next to Johnson as inspector Dan Clem opened the trunk. When Clem found white powder hidden in a wheel well, Ressam panicked and ran away. Ahmed Ressam did not hesitate for a second in choosing to flee rather than fight. For police officers worldwide, physical flight is a clear sign of guilt.

Officers intercepted Ressam as he tried to carjack a vehicle stopped at a nearby traffic light. Later it was determined that he had ties to Osama bin Laden, and had undergone terrorist training in Afghanistan in 1998. Ahmed was carrying bomb components, which he planned to assemble and detonate at California's Los Angeles International Airport (LAX).

After surveilling LAX ten months before his capture, Ressam planned to hide his bomb in a suitcase and set it off in a crowded passenger area on New Year's Eve. On April 6, 2001, Ahmed Ressam, the "Millennium Bomber," was convicted in Los Angeles in U.S. District Court of conspiracy to commit international terrorism, along with eight other criminal acts. He was sentenced to twenty-two years in prison. Had Ressam not appeared nervous and sweaty in December 1999, innocent lives may have been lost in his New Year's plot.

ANXIETY ALARM

Anxiety is a telltale sign that something is wrong. Eyes widen, fingers fidget, voices tremble, foreheads glisten with sweat. In his report to the FBI soon after September 11, 2001, Ken Boyer, owner of Boyer's Telecom Services in Springfield, Missouri, recounted how men of Middle Eastern background had asked to buy his turboprop Piper Saratoga for $500,000 (Doria and Menard 2001). "They wanted to buy it for cash that day. They meant business. There were no smiles or idle talk," Boyer said. The men appeared nervous, wore unkempt clothing, and were unshaven. They beseeched him in thickly accented English to sell the plane—for cash—right now. Crime signals told Boyer something was wrong, and he sounded the alarm to authorities.

BODY LANGUAGE IN AIRPORTS

In the United States, airport security used to be all about screening for weapons. Today it is also about screening for people with hostile intentions. While guns and explosives can be found with metal detectors and bomb-sniffing dogs, dangerous humans may be detected through behavior pattern recognition, or BPR. BPR is forensic code for watching body language.

On a March 2003 flight from Amsterdam to Minneapolis, leaving from the Netherlands' Schiphol Airport, my wife and I were questioned by a security screener who paid close attention to our demeanor. As he picked up my electric shaver and asked if I'd ever sent it out for service, his eyes searched mine for clues of uncertainty, nervousness, and deception. "No," I answered, with his gaze fastened to my face. The serious man in the dark uniform continued to stare from beneath his visored cap as he handled items in my kit bag.

The somber Dutchman was thorough, intimidating, and watchful. He certainly would have caught me had I lied. How different our treatment was at the beginning of our trip, in Seattle, where screeners searched our bags but not our faces. They looked for weapons, not BPR.

Raphael Ron, former security director at Ben-Gurion Airport in Israel, calls BPR the "human factor." "If you do not develop security procedures that go beyond technology," Ron insists, "you are doomed to lose at the end of the day" (Fickes 2003).

ON THE SAME TEAM

On December 21, 1969, three terrorists from the Popular Front for the Liberation of Palestine (PFLP) flew to Athens, Greece, to hijack a TWA plane and take it to Tunis. An airport clerk became suspicious when he saw each of them carrying exactly the same kind of baggage. Police opened the suitcases and found guns and explosives (O'Ballance 1979, 77–78). By carrying the same bags, the terrorists inadvertently announced that they were on the same team.

At U.S. airports in Boston, Chicago, Houston, Los Angeles, and other cities, police now train in techniques of behavior recognition. When officers see something suspicious, such as two passengers examining a restricted area, they engage them in conversation to detect anxiety or evasiveness. Stumbling answers, nervous hands stuffed into pockets, or evasive eyes could prompt a more thorough interrogation.

Had BPR been available at Dulles International Airport on September 11, 2001, screeners might have noted that not one of the al Qaeda terrorists who'd passed through security that day had looked at the guards. Years later, when TSA personnel viewed the 9/11 security tape, agents spotted the hijackers' downcast eyes. "They all looked away and had their heads down," one TSA analyst observed (Frank 2005b). On that fateful September morning, simultaneously averting the gaze from authorities might have been an actionable sign of hostile intentions.

HIS BEHAVIOR SET HIM APART

When one's mission in life is spectacularly different from those of everyone else, the visible behavior exhibited toward its completion tends to differ as well. I call this nonverbal principle the law of incongruous contrasts, and it especially applies to terrorists. When your goal is outlandish, the behavior you employ to achieve it appears outlandish, too. A case in point is the starkly incongruous demeanor—not in keeping with that which is correct, proper, or logical—of Zacarias Moussaoui, the French-Algerian terrorist.

In his highly publicized mug shot, Moussaoui's dark brown eyes stare straight ahead through lowered eyelids. His smooth, unwrinkled forehead is relaxed and untroubled; his lips in repose are untroubled as well. He wears a short goatee, and his head is shaved bald. In most societies, according to anthropologist Richard Alford, shaven heads "suggest an acceptance of discipline or order, denial or conformity" (Alford 1996, 7).

Moussaoui was called to arms in a dream; his mission in life was to hijack a jetliner and crash it into the U.S. White House. By any standard, this is an unusual goal. His spectacularly deviant mission led to some equally unusual behavior.

Moussaoui attended the Airman Flight School in Norman, Oklahoma, from February to May of 2001. Unlike most Airman students, he set himself apart spatially by refusing to live in school-provided housing. Unlike fellow enrollees, Moussaoui deceived those around him with conflicting accounts of his career goals. He told instructors he wanted to become a private pilot for rich Middle Eastern patrons. He told some students he had a pilot's job waiting in Chicago, and told others he wanted to fly for a living in England. Strangely, Zacarias Moussaoui had no previous experience flying airplanes, and his aptitude as a pilot was so low that the flight school was forced to ground him.

At odds with Moussaoui the man, Moussaoui's bizarre mission to blow up the White House put him in a most incongruous setting—professional flight school—in which the terrorist's behavior was bound to set him apart from the norm.

At their debriefing, pilot instructors described Mohammed Atta and other students who took part in the 9/11 attacks as being very "standoffish," former FBI profiler and special agent Joe Navarro reports in his book *Hunting Terrorists* (Navarro 2005, 50).

To further pursue his mission, in the summer of 2001 Moussaoui enrolled at a second institution, the Pan Am International Flight School in Eagan, Minnesota. There, the terrorist's demeanor seemed suspicious, once again, from the start. Instructors saw him as unusually uncooperative, insistent, and secretive. When asked about his personal life, Moussaoui was mysteriously evasive.

As at his first school, Moussaoui's behavior at Pan Am seemed palpably out of alignment. He paid for most of his $8,000 jumbo-jet flight simulator course in cash, with $100 bills. In a class on the Boeing 747 cockpit, Moussaoui's instructor, Clancy Prevost, saw right away that something was wrong. "He had no frame of reference whatsoever with a commercial airliner," Prevost said (Hirschkorn 2006).

When Prevost asked if Moussaoui was Muslim, Zacarias raised his voice and exclaimed, "I am nothing!" (Hirschkorn 2006). Moussaoui's angry tone of voice showed that Prevost's question had struck a nerve. Something about Moussaoui's ballistic vocal response seemed uncalled for. Like his evasive and uncooperative demeanor at the flight school, there was something about him that seemed suspicious, not quite right. Secretive, standoffish, deceptive, uncooperative, hotheaded—the signs piled up. Fortunately, Zacarias's anomalous behavior was not ignored by his trainers.

Considering the context—an unqualified pilot learning to fly a 747—on August 15, 2001, Pan Am contacted FBI officials in Minnesota. On August 17, agents arrested Moussaoui on charges of immigration violation to keep him in tow. Indicted in December 2001, Zacarias Moussaoui confessed in April 2005 to conspiring with al Qaeda in a plot to crash jetliners into U.S. landmarks. Had his unusual demeanor gone unnoticed, the terrorist might have succeeded.

A TALE OF TWO TERRORISTS

In contract work on video signals intelligence (SIGINT) for the U.S. Department of Defense in 2003, one of my assignments was to decode nonverbal signals, in publicly available videotapes, of the world's foremost terrorist, Osama bin Laden, and Iraqi president Saddam Hussein. Until then, few had studied their body language in a systematic way.

Osama bin Laden

Osama bin Laden, mastermind of the September 11, 2001, attacks on New York's World Trade Center and the Pentagon in Washington, D.C., was apparently injured shortly afterward. The injury came in December 2001, in Afghanistan, during the siege of Tora Bora. U.S. officials wanted to know if bin Laden was still mentally capable of leadership after the Tora Bora strike. In a thirty-three-minute videotape that aired December 27, 2001, on Al Jazeera television, shortly after the strike, bin Laden looked older, grayer, and physically weaker than he'd appeared in previous tapes. In this video—the last footage we were to see of him for years—bin Laden was gaunt, and the entire left side of his body seemed immobilized. Though left-handed, he made no gestures with his left arm, hand, or fingers.

From the tape—in which he listened and responded to others' comments without speaking himself—some saw in the silence and left-sided immobility evidence of a debilitating right-hemispheric stroke. If true, al Qaeda's top leader would no longer be able to lead. But from visible shrugs of his left shoulder, I concluded that he was neurologically intact. Had he incurred damage to the right side of his brain, as some inferred from the video, he'd be unable to raise, flex, or shrug his left shoulder.

Recall from chapter 2 that shoulders are mobile, jointed organs that connect the arms to the torso. The trapezius muscles that move them are linked to emotionally sensitive circuits of the accessory nerve (cranial XI). Had bin Laden suffered a cerebral stroke, these nerve links would have been cut and we would have seen no shrugs of his left shoulder. For me, seeing his shoulder shrug was like seeing a groundhog's shadow in winter: there would be many more months of terror.

Much is written about Osama bin Laden's religion and politics, but what is he like as a person? From videotapes and comments of eyewitnesses, we piece together a nonverbal profile of bin Laden the man.

His tall stature—six feet four to six feet five—and large hands suggest a leader in command. His slow, deliberate, thoughtful hand gestures reinforce the leadership image. Though shy, he is physically dominating. For a big man, Osama's body movements while walking, talking, and handling weapons are unhurried and poised. He seems capably in control.

For all the terror he's unleashed, bin Laden has been described as self-effacing, soft-spoken, mild-mannered, and polite. He dresses humbly, wears a plain white turban, and shares simple meals with seemingly adoring followers. It is said that he sometimes cooked for subordinates and worked alongside them on ordinary tasks. An anonymous source for PBS's *Frontline* wrote, "He speaks very little and looks serious most of the time. He would appear with a soft smile, but he seldom laughs."

How can a man with such an apparently benign demeanor be the world's most wanted terrorist? Judging from his body language, the answer lies in a dark inner core. Bin Laden's evil sentiments are revealed in a forty-minute videotape captured in 2001 in Jalalabad, Afghanistan. The candid video, released by the Pentagon on December 13, shows an unrehearsed scene of bin Laden smugly chuckling as he describes how his entire crew of 9/11 hijackers had died without knowing their true target until just before stepping onto the airplanes.

Using mime gestures to physically shape his thoughts—a stationary vertical hand depicted the skyscraper, a horizontal hand moving toward it represented a plane about to collide—bin Laden smiles a divulging, lighthearted grin as he speaks of the thousands of deaths he caused at the World Trade Center. After viewing the tape, New York mayor Rudy Giuliani said, "It leaves you wondering just how deep the evil of his heart and soul really is."

Just how deep is suggested by comparable body language of a notorious American serial killer, Ed Gein, whose lopsided grin showed when he talked of people who had recently died. Gein, the original "Psycho," after whom Alfred Hitchcock's 1960 thriller movie was named, had a habit of laughing at weirdly inappropriate times, "as though he were listening to some strange, private joke that no one else could hear" (Schechter 1989, 20). Belying his calm exterior, bin Laden's odd smile revealed an insidious wicked streak.

Saddam Hussein

The body language of Saddam Hussein is as telling as that of Osama bin Laden. When I received the Department of Defense's tape of CBS *60 Minutes II*'s interview with Saddam, I noticed a green UNCLASSIFIED sticker affixed to its back. The Q and A in Baghdad with Dan Rather had aired on national television on February 26, 2003, so the sticker seemed uncalled for. Millions saw the interview, and the question on everyone's mind that year had already echoed from nations around the world. Did Saddam— or did he not—have weapons of mass destruction? On July 9, 2003, I examined his body language for answers.

First, I did a word-for-word written transcript of Dan Rather's questions and Saddam's translated replies. Second, I inserted notations for Saddam Hussein's body language—every facial, hand, and body movement—below his verbal remarks. Notations include such behaviors as "closed mouth smile," "scratches left side of face," "looks off to left," "gazes down," "palms up," "palms down," and so on. Third, I attributed meanings to each body-language cue from definitions provided in *The Nonverbal Dictionary* (Givens 2003).

The study's fourth step was a semantic content analysis of themes and topics. I delineated seven major topics in the interview: (1) weapons of mass destruction (WMD), (2) asylum,

(3) bin Laden, (4) debate (Saddam wanted to debate President Bush on TV), (5) George Bush, (6) coffee, and (7) possible war in Iraq. Finally, in step five, I compared the body language within each of the seven topics, and concluded "from symptomatic arm gestures and facial expressions in his pre-war interview with Dan Rather, that Saddam Hussein was personally convinced he no longer had weapons of mass destruction."

Recall from chapters 1 and 2 that words may deceive, but the body cannot lie. For all but the best actors, lying is liable to show somewhere in facial or body movements, and likely in both. After careful observation of Saddam Hussein, I saw no visible deception in his expressions, gestures, or movements. His body language while discussing the benign topic coffee did not significantly differ from the more arousing topic WMD.

Indeed, Saddam's body language when he said, "Americans like coffee" was the same as when he said, "These missiles have been destroyed." I detected no significant stimulation of his sympathetic nervous system in either topic. Had he been polygraphed, I believe he would have tested negative for lying.

Saddam Hussein's words were congruous with his actions. "Americans like coffee"; "These missiles have been destroyed": in Saddam's mind, neither statement was a lie. He was personally convinced that both statements were true. According to his body language, there were no WMD in Iraq.

On March 20, 2003, the U.S. invasion of Iraq commenced at approximately 02:30 UTC (Coordinated Universal Time). In a speech on April 25, 2003, President George Bush called Saddam's WMD "a threat to Americans." On March 2, 2004, United Nations weapons inspectors agreed there were no WMD in Iraq. On January 12, 2005, almost two years after President Bush had ordered the invasion, U.S. officials called off their search for Iraqi

SADDAM'S BODY LANGUAGE

After his capture by American forces on December 13, 2003, many commented on Iraqi dictator Saddam Hussein's body language. "I found a very broken man. . . . His body language showed that he was very miserable," said Muwaffaq al-Rubaiye, a member of the Iraqi Governing Council, shortly after Saddam's arrest (Anonymous 2003b).

Atlanta-based body-language expert Patti Wood told BBC News that Saddam pointed his fingers while speaking, as if to attack his enemies, sliced the air with his pen used as a "symbolic sword," joined his fingertips together to display the power-connoting "steeple" gesture, and stared at interviewers to frighten them (Anonymous 2004).

On trial in Baghdad for ordering the killing of more than 140 people in Dujail in 1982, Saddam made loud, defiant outbursts throughout the proceedings. He repeatedly pointed his stiffened forefinger at the judge, defiantly pounded his fists for emphasis as he spoke, and showed exasperation, impatience, and nervousness on his face. When angry, his face turned red, his eyes twitched, and his heavy lids opened widely. At times he fully extended both arms and aimed fisted hands at the judge, an intention movement for physically striking.

Overall, Saddam Hussein's body language reflected someone who felt self-important, revengeful, fearful, arrogant, and aloof—the body language of a thoroughly unrepentant criminal.

WMD. Our conclusion, based on Saddam's nonverbal behavior, was apparently correct.

A terrorist's crime signals send explicit messages of fear on behalf of personal, religious, or revolutionary goals. Since a terrorist's mission in life is spectacularly different from everyone else's, his behavior is visibly different as well. Terrorists stand out because, as the law of incongruous contrasts predicts, when one's goal is outlandish, the behavior employed to achieve it also appears outlandish. Here are some transparent warnings that a suspicious person could be more than just your average creepy criminal:

- On a plane, behavior counter to your "experiential blueprint" of what's normal
- At a national border, people walking in line "on a mission" instead of side by side
- Sweating, hemming, hawing, and dawdling at customs checkpoints
- Avoiding inspectors' eyes at airport security
- Outlandish behavior toward an outlandish goal
- Inappropriate bags or backpacks carried into a crowd
- Suspicious surveillance of passageways in public places

In the next chapter, you will learn to decipher the body language of minor-league terrorists known as street gangs. Though not likely to use explosives, radioactive materials, or poison gas, gangs still merit your closest attention.

8

READING THE GANG SIGNS

The more flamboyant the clothing, the better.

—A self-designated gangster

IN THE SPRING OF 2006, from my hidden vantage point just up the street, I made field observations of two wannabe street-gang members acting out in front of their suburban home. They are brothers, both seventeen. "Sid" and "Homey" belong to a loose confederation of young men Spokane police officers would call a "hybrid gang." Hybrid gang members come from different neighborhoods of the city, wear different colors, and include boys from different ethnic backgrounds.

Each day, Sid and Homey walk out their front door sometime between 11:00 a.m. and noon. From waist to knees, their loose khaki clothing looks more like skirt than pants. The boys literally waddle in fabric, pace back and forth on the lawn, check cell phones, smoke cigarettes, and spit. They rotate their oversize caps and make jerky hand gestures as they speak. Over and over again, they spit.

Girls who visit Sid and Homey on the family front lawn never spit. Visiting boys in the same style of clothing always do. They jerk their heads insolently sideward, bringing attention to themselves with the erratic head movement. It sends an aggressive message about territory that seems to say, "What I spit on, I own." Spitting also shows, since the boys spit with each other in syncopated rhythm, that they're on the same team.

As they walk together to and fro on the sidewalk, penguinlike, the boys self-consciously adjust their trousers. They strategically pull down their khaki pants to display boxer shorts beneath. The boxer shorts are usually plaid, often colorful, and worn to catch the eye. The boys' repeated exhibitionistic lowering of their trousers and shorts is a ritual replete with meaning. In a somewhat dubious reading, the display is thought to suggest or allude to prison sex. I read the display more straightforwardly, as a way of showing gang solidarity by mimicking each other's actions and disrespectfully mooning the powers that be. Showing their shorts simultaneously bonds the boys and signals disrespect for authority.

When Sid and Homey's dad isn't home, cars with boom boxes pull up alongside the grassy parking strip. Usually, a boy wearing an extralarge baseball cap and baggy pants gets out as comrades stay in the idling vehicle. I hear the thumping, boom-boom noise announcing, "We are here." The delivery boy carries a black gym bag up to the front door and enters the brothers' two-story home. I can't see inside, but soon he returns with the bag and gets back in the car. Is he delivering or receiving drugs? Do drugs and money actually change hands? I can't see.

When the gang's not around, Sid and Homey never look happy. They seem chronically annoyed. They never go to school. They never mow the lawn. That's Dad's job. Homey and Sid don't have jobs, unless it's selling narcotics. From my vantage point up the street, I can't tell. But I can tell from their dad's demeanor and tone of voice that he wishes they'd do something more productive with their lives. Soon they'll be eighteen, legal adults, and the gang will be all they have. I never talked to the brothers, but from their non-verbal actions I predict that these wannabes are gangster gonna-bes.

DECIPHERING GANG HATS

Criminals often camouflage their actions to blend into the wood-work, but street gangs boldly proclaim their identity with graffiti, hand gestures, tattoos, bandannas, haircuts, and "bling" (jew-elry). Like wasps, skunks, and coral snakes, gang members wear conspicuous, high-contrast, aposematic warning marks, clothing, and coloration to deter rivals. A favorite combination is primary yellow on jet black—to human eyes the most visible of all color blends—to suggest, like a coiled serpent, "Don't tread on me!"

Hats have long been favored signs of gang membership. In the 1850s, members of New York City's Plug Uglies gang wore large plug hats—bowlers or top hats—stuffed with leather, rags, and wool scraps. Like helmets, the padded hats protected heads in gang fights, and announced gang affiliation on the streets. Plug Uglies wore hobnail boots, carried bricks and clubs in their hands, and stuck pistols in their belts. But the looming hats de-fined them and proclaimed their identity from afar.

Gang hats are expressive today. Members of the Black Gang-ster Disciples, a Chicago-based street gang, wear baseball caps with brims angled to the right. In Los Angeles, members of the Bloods gang wear red caps, while rival Crips wear blue. New York City's Black Pearls wear large, soft-brimmed, purple-and-white hats for identity, while members of the Turbans gang wear black caps with showy gold pom-poms.

For gang members, wearing the same hat shows unity. Caps often display emblems of professional ball clubs, but in a deeper sense the group they refer to is the boys in the gang. Unlike women's hats, which are designed to show individuality, men's hats are part of a uniform to show membership on a team. This explains the generally standardized design of turbans, fedoras, fezzes, and the gang members' signature caps.

> ### THUGZ
>
> The English word "thug" comes from Sanskrit *sthagayati,* "to cover or conceal." Indian "Thugz" were professional criminals and assassins who pillaged towns in northern India eight hundred years ago. Like modern street gangs, Thugz used identifying hand gestures, clothing signals, and symbolic rituals to recognize one another and to frighten victims at the same time.

DANCES WITH FOES

Gang identity may be displayed in shoes as well. Shoes with the right-hand tongue curled up and the left curled down, or vice versa, and with the shoelaces tied up to only five holes, or only to six, can also show membership in a gang. Members of the Gangster Disciples, one of the biggest street gangs in the nation according to U.S. Department of Justice figures, wear black and blue laces to proclaim their identity. On the street, such seemingly minor messages have major meanings. Misreading a shoe may be hazardous to your health.

Feet, too, can warn. In the conspicuous "pimp strut," men drag one foot behind and "limp" from side to side. The gang member's warning limp evolved from a widespread stepping style called the "swagger walk." The swagger walk is a masculine gait boys and men use to appear deceptively "bigger" through exaggerated side-to-side movements in their stride. To widen personal territory, they strut to fill the space on either side of their bodies with movement. The strutting motion connotes greater weight and stature as the walker seems to take up more room on the street.

The swagger walk may have a recent origin in the American South, where prison work crews rhythmically trod together in chain gangs along county roads. It therefore harks back to Southern slavery, and persists today in rap, rock, and heavy metal music. In their 1991 album *Slave to the Grind*, for instance, Skid Row's hit song, "Livin' on a Chain Gang," was praised by one reviewer for its "hellish swagger." Yet the swagger walk itself is actually ancient, with roots in primate displays designed to make the upper body loom larger.

Properly walked down a sidewalk, a gangster's swagger projects an aura of power and dominance. The walk is not generally used to greet women. It is performed instead as men enter taverns or bars to announce their presence to rival males or potential girlfriends inside. The best-known swagger walk belonged not to a gangster, however, but to good-guy actor John Wayne, who starred in such movie classics as *Rio Bravo* (1959), *The Alamo* (1960), and *True Grit* (1970). That John Wayne seemed larger than life on the screen was due less to his six-feet-four stature than to his swagger.

Like gangsters, our closest animal relatives, the great apes, show dominance by straightening and holding their arms outward, away from the body, as they swagger-walk from side to side. For additional clout, gorillas add chest pounding to the display.

In the 1970s, members of youth gangs added power to persona with martial-arts movements and dance steps. Rivals showed off with jumping, cutting, diving, and head-spinning routines of competitive break dancing. Their aggressive dance moves signified who had ascendancy on the street. Break dancing began in New York street gangs in violent body work shaped from East Coast "uprock," West Coast "locking," and stylistic kung fu practice routines. The exaggerated body language of break dance showcased athleticism, balance, and strength in motions that were both entertaining and scary to watch.

In the early days of break dance, young hoodlums used battle-oriented movements and gestures to show rivals—in clear nonverbal terms—that they stood little chance of winning a fight. In Brooklyn and the South Bronx, some gangs used the break-dance ritual as a symbolic substitute for brawling itself. Before a rumble, disputing gangs met to show each other, through mock-contact gestures, what they faced in the upcoming battle. In rare cases, events on the dance floor ignited genuine combat with weapons and fists.

After intense media attention, the threatening body language of break dance evolved away from gangs to popular youth culture as a form of entertainment. Singer Michael Jackson's moonwalk is a case in point. The gravity-defying dance step premiered in 1983 in a performance of his best-selling album *Thriller* (1982). Jackson unwittingly touched off a fascination with the body language of street gangs that continues to this day. First popularized in *West Side Story* (1961), gang signals attained star quality in *Thriller*.

Another dance that emerged from gang life is the stylized martial-art form of capoeira. Far older than break dance, capoeira was practiced by sixteenth-century African slaves in Brazil. When slavery ended there in 1888, criminal gangs of

Afro-Brazilian men practiced the dance's acrobatic moves—kicks, jumps, spins, cartwheels, headstands, handstands, and elbow strikes—to enhance group solidarity and terrorize any who would stand in their way. Like break dance, the athletic moves of capoeira are largely symbolic. Rather than delivering an actual blow, they suggest the possibility or capability of striking. Encoded in both of these gang-inspired dance routines is a militant warning about superiority in battle.

GANGSTER SEE, GANGSTER DO

In the underworld of crime, gangsters are the most imitative of all criminals. They wear the same hats, hairstyles, apparel, accessories, and footwear as their fellow gang members. They sport the same tattoos on the same body parts, wear the same bandannas, and carry the same weapons as toted by peers. The same hand signals are used in the same spaces, places, and situations, by the same people, over and over, with little change for years. If imitation is the sincerest form of flattery, gangs most sincerely flatter themselves.

For many a hoodlum—and for wannabes who emulate them—the uniform begins with voluminous khaki pants, several sizes too big and with a low inseam, at knee level or below. The pants are worn loose and low on the hips to expose underwear, and to figuratively thumb the nose at parents and authorities. Police like the baggies because they make it harder for criminals to run fast or jump over fences to escape.

Next on is an oversize T-shirt, which also hangs low, then a pair of shiny white athletic shoes. An immense puffy jacket goes on, topped by an oversize NBA cap with a signature wide brim. On the sidewalk, you notice the gangster's slow shuffle with the upper body tilting side to side as he walks. You see hands pulling at pants, bouts of gratuitous spitting, and eyes affixed to a cell phone.

In his book *Gangsta in the House*, Houston police officer Mike Knox described the look in 1995: "What is this 'look'? You know already: the extremely baggy pants, worn so low on the hips as to barely cover the buttocks—exposing one's underwear; the super-extra-large shirt, two-sizes-too-big shoes, hat on backward (or sideways or upside down); no-bones-in-the-body kind of walk that many youths believe cool or 'fresh' or 'hype'" (Knox 1995, 80). A decade later, for many street gangs the look is still the same.

SAGGING PANTS

From the oficial Web site of the Los Angeles Police Department, February 11, 2007: Gang clothing styles can be easily detected because of the specific way gang members wear their clothing. Examples are preferences for wearing baggy or 'sagging' pants or having baseball caps turned at an angle. Gang members often prefer particular brands of shoes, pants or shirts. For example, some gangs like to wear plaid shirts in either blue, brown, black or red. These shirts are worn loosely and untucked. Gang graffiti, symbols, messages or gang names can be written or embroidered on jackets, pants and baseball caps. Other identifying items include belt buckles with the gang's initials, key chains, starter jackets (team jackets), and red or blue bandannas commonly called 'rags.'

It's all for show. Whether in a gang or not, the young man's complex body language—the billowing costume and puffed-up demeanor—is meant to defy authority, suggest gang affiliation, bluff rivals, and attract members of the opposite sex—all at the same time.

Recognizing how the body language of gang members differs from wannabes who mimic their actions is a good way to protect yourself from harm. In nature, harmless animals may mimic the movements, patterns, and colors of toxic species. Looking, acting, and sounding more dangerous than they are helps bluff predators away. The eastern coral snake (*Micrurus fulvius*), for example, is a beautiful, highly venomous serpent with aposematic color bands of red, yellow, and black. Each red band is bracketed by yellow.

Meanwhile, the harmless, nonvenomous scarlet king snake (*Lampropeltis triangulum*) has look-alike bands of red, yellow, and black, but each red band is bounded on either side by black. Mimicking danger signs of the coral snake helps the wannabe king snake keep predators at bay. Biologists advise that you recognize color patterns to help save your life. As the saying warns, "Red and yellow kills a fellow—red and black, friend of Jack."

True gang members emulate one another not only by dressing alike but by wearing equivalent tattoos. Their designs are not as artistic as the elegant, needled images available in a hygienic tattoo parlor. Bloods, for example, may spell out "blood" one crude letter at a time across the fingers of a right hand (they favor signaling on the right). "RBD," for Red Blood Dragons, may be roughly tattooed in blue letters down a forearm.

Crips tattoo names, nicknames, and local chapters across their chests or down their left upper arms (they signal to the left). Affiliated with the Crips, Oriental Loks wear Old English script tattoos across the length of both forearms. Hispanic gangs often wear tattoos on their bellies, necks, backs, legs, forearms, upper arms, and hands. Three dots grouped in a triangle, tattooed almost anywhere on the body, is symbolism for *Mi Vida Loca*—"My Crazy Life."

Gangland tattoos are more functional than artistic. They're for affiliation rather than adornment. Street gang tattoos are often blurry, indistinct, and monochromatic. Rather than artful images, numbers (a "5," for instance, in the middle of a five-pointed star) and letters in cursive, Old English, or Gothic script are used. Committed gang members tattoo on their hands, necks, and faces—on body areas not covered by cloth. Emulators, on the other hand, rarely wear gang tattoos and almost never tattoo on the body's exposed parts.

Another way to tell gangsters from imitators is through hand movements. Mimics may use palm-down rap gestures as they speak, but rarely use the crooked, contorted, complex, symbolically coded hand-and-finger movements of organized street gangs. The latter's hand signals take practice to master and have functional use on the street, both to show gang membership and to challenge those who would trespass.

Manual signs may be flashed for numbers, letters, and words. Crips sign the letter "C," for example, along with a number signifying their neighborhood or street (Sachs 1997). Many gangs use alphabetic signals borrowed from American Sign Language for the deaf, or ASL. Unaffiliated mimics, who wear the gangster look to high school but don't belong to a gang, have little need to practice ASL or display the intricate finger positions of Imperial Gangsters or Maniac Latin Disciples. For a mimic, displaying underpants is enough.

The visual credo of "Gangster see, gangster do" is rooted in the reptilian principle of isopraxism. "Isopraxism" is the scientific name for an imitative response identified in 1975 by neuroanatomist Paul MacLean. In Greek, *iso* is "same" and *praxis* means "behavior." Isopraxism is a biologically inspired tendency to mimic, which leads gangsters to copy, emulate, and repeat the actions of respected peers. MacLean located the imitation response in a primitive motor center of the forebrain called the basal ganglia.

Isopraxism explains why gang members dress alike and adopt the same body language, gestures, and voice tones. Wearing the same baggy pants and the same NBA cap to look alike suggests that they think and feel alike as well. In animals, isopraxism shows in the simultaneous head nodding of lizards, in the group gobbling of turkeys, and in the synchronous preening of birds. Gang members show isopraxic movements, colors, and adornment from their heads to their toes to stay socially connected and psychologically united.

GANGSTER GARB

The visual theme of gang membership is to stand out clearly as a gangster. In the 1940s, Chicago mobsters wore navy pin-striped, double-breasted suits with very wide, peaked lapels, double-pleated trousers, and wide cuffs. Jackets had tapered-waist fits and wide shoulders. Worn beneath jackets, tight-fitting, high-buttoned vests with satin backs and adjusters gave a serious look.

Earlier, in the 1930s, a Los Angeles gangster might have worn a "zoot suit." It, too, had a wide-shouldered, narrow-waisted look. The very long jacket, double-breasted with peaked lapels, gave a loose and casual drape. Its hem dropped well below the wearer's dangled fingertips. Fuller-fitting, baggy pleated pants were worn with a showy taper from the knee down. Accessories included suspenders, a glittering zoot chain, a very thin snake or crocodile belt, and a fedora with turned-down brim and pinch front crown. Conspicuous two-tone oxford or "spectator" shoes completed the message: "Notice me."

THREE-DOG PLIGHT

I was enjoying a midsummer's brunch at the Park Bench Café in Spokane's leafy Manito Park when a blue Buick sedan on the street caught my eye. From my outside table, I noticed the car moving toward me at the unusually slow speed of five miles per hour.

As the vehicle neared, I saw animated body movements within. Three male heads bobbed up and down and turned—in synchrony—toward a young boy on a bicycle pedaling beside them. Suddenly, a black cylinder pushed out the opened rear window on the driver's side. The teenagers' heads kept bobbing, and I saw openmouthed smiles and heard laughter as the cylinder took aim, then fired at the unsuspecting boy on his bike.

What I'd witnessed that sunny day was a drive-by shooting. Luckily the "gun" was an ISG—an improvised squirt gun—made with vinyl tubing attached to a water balloon. The damage was slight, a soaked T-shirt and the boy's wounded pride. The assailants' heads kept bobbing as they laughed, and then their faces snapped forward in unison to stare straight ahead as the blue sedan sped off. No real harm done, and I casually resumed my brunch.

Though a minor occurrence, this proto-drive-by is in some ways a reflection of major violence. I call it a "proto" drive-by because the squirt-gun snipers serve as a model for attacks with real handguns and live ammunition. Take the central fact that three teenage boys were involved. I liken their badgering to the pack behavior of *Canis familiaris*, the domestic dog. When you see one dog loose on the street, you take notice. When you see two dogs, you take care before stepping past. When you see three dogs, you take cover. Three boys in a slow-moving sedan are like three loose dogs on the street. The volatile pack mentality emerges in both triads.

Biologists explain pack mentality as a form of group mobbing called "aggression out." When two or more animals focus aggression on an outside victim, they feel psychologically closer and allied. Bonds between them gel as they join in mobbing. Group laughter, like what I'd seen in the blue Buick, is a perfect example of aggression out. The boys' laughing vocalizations sounded like the mobbing calls biologists record in free-ranging monkeys and apes.

As the squirt-gun gang sped away, I realized I actually knew them. They were high school seniors whom I had met. One was an Eagle Scout. By themselves, each was trustworthy, kind, and morally straight. But together on that summer day they'd formed a pack. Three teenage boys bouncing around in a slow-moving vehicle is a clear and present warning sign of mischief or—as we'll see below—danger.

FROM SQUIRT GUN TO SHOTGUN

If body language in a water-pistol strike includes animated bouncing, laughing, and group mobbing, what does a real drive-by look like? To compare squirt guns with shotguns, we consider the court documents and chronology pieced together on a gang-related drive-by in San Antonio, Texas, in which two juvenile gang members planned and perpetrated a fatal shooting at a rival gangster's house (Anonymous 1998).

The scene opens on the night of January 30, 1994, with friends "Oscar" and "Noel" plotting mobile mayhem in a car parked outside Oscar's home. Oscar walks into his house to get a rifle while Noel sits and waits in the car. To keep from being seen with a gun, Oscar carries the firearm out through his bedroom window. Back in the car, Oscar tells Noel, "You are the one that wants to do it," and gives him the rifle.

Noel has never seen the gun before. It is the first gun he's ever used. The look and feel of the weapon make the aggressive act they plan to unleash on rival gang member "Manuel" seem palpably more real now than just a plan. As Oscar drives with Noel sitting beside him, the boys talk about how to do the shooting.

Noel loads the gun with seven bullets. Clearly, it is not a squirt gun. "I don't know what kind of bullets they were," Noel will later say, "but they were real long."

Oscar drives from his house to the victim's house to see if anyone is home. They see shadows of people walking inside. Oscar slowly drives to the back of the house, where Noel sits in his passenger door's open window, legs inside the vehicle with his upper body perched outside. As Oscar keeps the motor running for a fast getaway, Noel fires over the vehicle's roof into the house. That there are two in the mob squad makes shooting easier than if Noel had acted alone.

After the initial volley, Oscar drives to the front, where Noel shoots twice more. On his final firing, Noel aims at a sliding glass door. Hearing nothing, he doesn't know if he's hit it or not. Oscar anxiously drives away and then turns on the headlights without waiting to assess the damage. He drives back to his own home and returns the gun, as he took it, furtively through his bedroom window. When Oscar reappears he drives them to yet another home, that of Noel's cousin "Marta."

As they go in, Noel starts crying. Oscar tells him, "You're just like that because it's your first time." After a ten-minute stay at Marta's, Oscar drives Noel back to the house where their plot commenced. Oscar tells Noel not to say anything to anybody—"to nobody or else our asses are going down."

The targets of the boys' drive-by saw no crime signals beforehand. Since it was dark, and they were inside, nobody spotted the slow-moving vehicle with teenage boys aboard. According to court records, victims testified that they heard two rounds of gunshots that night (Anonymous 1998). The first came from the back of the house. During the second shooting phase, in front, shots hit the walls of the house. Soon after the gunfire ceased, an occupant found her four-year-old grandson pinned against the wall, bleeding from his head. Later the grandson, Raymundo, died from his wound.

In court, Marta testified that the juvenile gangsters looked "nervous and hyper" when they returned, telling her they'd shot at the house. The boys soon left, after stating they were going back to check the fruits of their aggression-out shooting spree at rival Manuel's. Returning then a second time to Marta's, the boys again looked hyperactive and nervous as they told her they'd shot up the house one more time.

A few days after the January drive-by, Noel confessed to teachers at his Brentwood Middle School. San Antonio police were called to investigate. Noel told them he'd been sick and unable to sleep since the shooting. Police described Noel's demeanor as "polite, remorseful, and very upset" (Dawson 1999). Later, on December 30, 1998, Noel and Oscar were found guilty of capital murder.

The body language of both attacks, with the squirt gun and the real gun, looked fundamentally the same. Excitable teenage boys in slow-moving vehicles egged each other on with ritualized mobbing and targeted aggression out. Had they acted alone, it's possible nothing would have happened in either case. In gangland, it takes a pack to attack.

AUTHORITY, GO FIGURE

If gang signals are shaped by ostentation, imitation, and aggression out, they are fanned by authority. In gangs you must do what you're told. From a nonverbal perspective, the imperative to follow the leader goes deeper than orders issued in words. To probe the body language of gang authority, we look at court records of a brutal kidnapping case that involved members of Chicago's oldest black street gang, the Vice Lords.

To greet each other, members bend their fingers and thumbs into coded "VL" shapes. According to the official Vice Lord Manifesto, "Failure to carry out an order promptly and efficiently could endanger the life of yourself or other Vice Lords" (Sachs 1997, 158). In other words, you must always do what you're told. As in many street gangs, the Vice Lord chain of command begins with a small cadre of authority figures, "generals" and "chiefs," who tell others, the "foot soldiers," what to do.

ON AUTHORITY OF CHARLES MANSON

On April 19, 1971, Charles Manson, leader of the notorious Manson Family, was sentenced to die for orchestrating the first-degree murder of actress Sharon Tate and others killed in the 1969 Los Angeles area massacre known as the Tate-LaBianca murders. In 1972, the California Supreme Court abolished the state's death penalty, and Manson is serving a life sentence without possibility of parole.

Manson used repetition to program gang members' minds. Like Adolf Hitler, he repeated the same phrases over and over again, "on almost a daily basis," to overcome inhibitions to his evil philosophy and plans (Bugliosi 1974, 627). Also as with Hitler, followers described Manson's eyes as "hypnotic" (Bugliosi 1974, 615). To isolate his disciples, Manson allowed no clocks or newspapers in the group's home. He used isopraxism—group activities such as communal cooking, cleaning, and sewing—to unite the group as a gang. After uniting his gangsters as "family," Manson programmed them to kill.

On June 15, 1993, Paloy Finnie was at work in the Gannes Beauty Shop in Memphis, Tennessee. Fatefully, Charles Thompson, a Vice Lord chief, approached and asked for the whereabouts of Finnie's sister. The sister, Torshia Burks, had reportedly been

Thompson's live-in girlfriend (Anonymous 2000b). Paloy Finnie answered that he didn't know, and Thompson left.

Minutes later, Charles Thompson returned with his brother Derrick. Charles asked again about the whereabouts of Finnie's sister. When Finnie repeated that he didn't know, the Thompson brothers abducted him to a third brother's home and proceeded to beat him. Afterward they drove Finnie, with a sheet covering his head, to their sister's home, where, on June 16, he was severely beaten for two hours with a tire iron, a water hose, pipes, and fists.

Vice Lord chief Charles Thompson—aided by Vice Lords Derrick Thompson, Marcus Daniels, and Derrick Vernon—finally released Finnie onto the street, with a swollen face, a broken right elbow, cracked ribs, cuts on his left arm, burn marks on his skin, and pain throughout his body.

At sentencing, the trial court indicated that "Mr. [Charles] Thompson was the one that was directing the action. And these men were carrying it out." The judge concluded that Vice Lord Derrick Vernon was "apparently obeying the dictates of the chief."

Vice Lord chief Charles Thompson led by the dictates of his body language. He hit the victim, on his own authority, and his foot soldiers joined in the mobbing. No corporate memo changed hands. His was leadership by example: Gangster see, gangster do.

> **Vice Lord chief Charles Thompson led by the dictates of his body language.**

Colors worn by Vice Lords are gold, black, and red. Team clothing—a University of Nevada, Las Vegas (UNLV), sweatshirt, a Chicago Bulls T-shirt, or a Chicago Blackhawks red-and-black jacket—shows membership through colors and letters

(UNLV backward signifies "Vice Lords Nation United"). Additionally, members wear tattoos of the five-pointed star and spray-paint graffiti images of top hats on neighborhood walls. These are all visual components of the Vice Lord uniform.

We understand the role uniforms play in authority from a famous simulation study of prison life conducted in 1971 at Stanford University. With the donning of an authority-connoting uniform, power suffuses a person. In Philip G. Zimbardo's pioneering experiment, students were randomly assigned roles of either guard or prisoner in a mock prison convincingly staged in a campus basement.

Uniformed guards wore khaki military shirts with button-flap pockets and shoulder straps designed to make the upper body look bigger. Khaki pants worn with thick black belts and black boots reinforced the display. Mirror sunglasses dehumanized prisoners by withholding personal eye contact. Guards carried billy clubs to suggest authority bolstered by the possibility of physical strikes.

Meanwhile, prisoners wore formless white dresslike smocks without underclothes. Observers noted that the prisoners dressed in smocks without underwear walked and sat submissively, more like women than men. Prisoners also wore rubber sandals, which destabilized their bodily stance, and covered their hair with women's nylon stocking caps. The psychic damage done to the prisoners by the uniformed guards was so disturbing that the study, which was scheduled to last two weeks, was canceled after just six days.

Like the Vice Lords, who dressed in physical and psychic uniforms of the day, Zimbardo's guards abused prisoners from the united front of their uniforms. Fanned by their leaders—the Vice Lord chief, Thompson, and an abusive guard the prisoners called "John Wayne"—the power instilled by their attire was directed outward toward helpless victims. In both the street and the prison-guard gangs, ritualized mobbing is inflamed by the uniformity of their look. The gangsters simply do what they saw others do.

Seeing gang signals, the best strategy is avoidance. Avoid gang involvement as you would avoid contact with poisonous wasps, coral snakes, or rattlers. When you see illegal acts, report them. Since you are one and gang members are many, do not step in by yourself. A growing number of police departments now have gang-control units, with officers trained to respond to the idiosyncratic habits, movements, fashion statements, and body language of street gangs.

Here is a short list of signs that a person might be more threatening than your average wannabe gangster:

- Shows up with friends wearing color-coded caps and shoelaces
- Wears a crude, monochromatic tattoo on his neck
- Defiantly spits in public, monitors surroundings, and exhibits nervous, stressed, hyperactive demeanor
- Seems abnormally self-absorbed in own peer group
- Uses enigmatic hand gestures with peers

In the next chapter, you will learn to decipher the body language of corporate gangsters—people who abuse their power to commit white-collar crime.

9

CORRUPT BUSINESS DESIGNS

Everyone who practices evil hates the light.

—JOHN 3:20-21

IF STREET GANGS are flamboyant in dress, dance, tattoos, and body language, corporate wrongdoers stay buttoned down and muted behind the scenes. Each morning they shower, don business suits, and disappear into cubicles or offices behind closed doors. Perpetrators of white-collar crimes—from insider trading to securities fraud—are often anonymous, invisible, and faceless.

Faceless, that is, until the U.S. Department of Justice shines a light on their greed. As public knowledge surfaces about wrongdoings at Enron, Pfizer, and Arthur Andersen—and by such billionaire moguls as Martha Stewart—a curious portrait emerges of corporate kinesics at the highest levels of power.

Far from being faceless, leaders of big companies actually make faces—pout, frown, clench their jaws in anger, and give looks that could kill. They overstep office boundaries, stand too close in hallways, shout, scream, and lift supercilious eyebrows in wrathful scorn. In the workplace, imperious demeanor is a warning sign. Confrontational body language shows that corruption may be at hand. Employers who aggressively act out could be one step away from breaking the law—or may have done so already.

What do Ivan Boesky, Andrew Fastow, and Martha Stewart have in common? Each has been a corporate mogul, each was known as a bullying boss, and each has been convicted of white-collar crimes. Prior to stepping over the legal line, each employer suffered a loss of anger control and engaged in the juvenile behavior of schoolyard bullies.

Junk-bond dealer and financial wizard Ivan ("I think greed is healthy") Boesky routinely screamed at staffers on the job. An able bully in his own right, Andrew Fastow, former chief financial officer at Enron, has been called hotheaded, brutally ambitious, and deeply insecure. Media maven Martha Stewart has been described as a chronic bully in the workplace. Convicted of conspiracy, making false statements, and obstructing justice, Stewart was designated by one of her staffers as "the boss from hell."

Criminal bosses abuse power in the workplace much as bullies abuse victims on the playground. Lacking empathy and social skills, bullies grab for control behaviorally through fisted gestures, glaring eyes, and humiliating tones of voice. Bullying bosses create a toxic atmosphere that breeds fear, resentment, and low morale. The more they dominate, the more their power grows. And soon, peering down imperial noses from on high, the line between good and evil looks thin enough to step over with impunity.

Criminal bosses abuse power in the workplace much as bullies abuse victims on the playground.

IMPERIAL MARTHA

One who stepped over the line was billionaire and former CEO of Martha Stewart Living Omnimedia, Martha H. Stewart. On March 5, 2004, a federal jury found Stewart, then sixty-two, guilty on four counts of obstructing justice and lying to investigators about the sale of her ImClone Systems stock on December 27, 2001. According to *USA Today*, Martha showed a "stoic, expressionless face" throughout the six-week trial. A behavioral sign of nondenial denial, showing no emotion in court strongly suggests guilt. According to CNN, Martha showed no emotion when the verdict was read, and was "poker-faced" as she left the courtroom. From televised news clips, I watched Martha's lips tighten on the courthouse steps just after the trial as her public smile gave way to a disgruntled frown.

On July 16, 2004, Martha Stewart was sentenced to five months in prison and fined $30,000. Speaking outside the courthouse after sentencing, her mouth's depressor anguli oris muscles again contracted to pull her lip corners visibly down. Then, in her trademark husky voice, Stewart vowed, "I'll be back."

Martha Stewart stepped over the legal line three times. First, she sold nearly four thousand shares of her ImClone stock after allegedly learning from insiders that its value was about to plunge. Second, she told investors in her company that she was innocent, in part, reportedly, to keep them from unloading their Martha Stewart Living Omnimedia stock. And third, she lied about her actions to federal investigators, which led to the four-felony conviction.

There were no obvious signs of criminality beforehand. But to the trained observer there were subtle—and not so subtle—crime signals. In the secretive world of white-collar crime, offenses take place privately—behind closed doors, on paper, in e-mails, and over the phone. Stewart's ImClone stock sale was initially confidential. Suspicions were raised after the federal government arrested ImClone's founder, Sam Waksal, on charges of insider trading. Subsequent investigation revealed that prior to making her sale, Stewart had allegedly been tipped by insiders linked to Waksal. Had he not been charged, her offense would probably have gone unnoticed.

How could a woman of Martha Stewart's public stature become a convicted felon? Judging from body language before and after the crime, stature itself was to blame. Throughout her career from model to stockbroker, from caterer to TV star to conglomerate CEO, Martha Stewart's immutable corporate goal has been to inflate her stature. How does that manifest itself in nonverbal demeanor and body language? Physically, stature is the height of a body in an upright position. Socially, stature is an achieved or ascribed level of status within a community. Nonverbally, both may be exaggerated. Martha Stewart was a genius at inflating her corporate size through an array of body movements, postures, and voice qualities that made her seem bigger than she really was. Her deep voice, belittling speech tones, and dismissive gestures were all tools intended to make others feel small.

According to Christopher Byron, author of *Martha Inc.*, Stewart summarily ended conversations with underlings by walking away or by hanging up the telephone without saying goodbye. She controlled the timing and dismissed them at will.

Martha managed colleagues by treating them "authoritatively," and came across as "bossy" and "arrogant." Control reverberated in her voice tones, and those who interrupted her risked "tongue-lashings." As Byron wrote, "She answered her phone with a single barked question: 'What?'" (Byron 2002, 299).

He reported that employees "lived in fear" of crossing paths with Martha Stewart in the company hallway. She sometimes seemed pleasant, but at other times would "scream at people and berate them in public" (Byron 2002, 300). Which way she'd act was anybody's guess. At one meeting, Martha threw a coffee cup against the wall and shouted, "How come everyone is so stupid around here?" (Byron 2002, 307).

Tone of voice reflects how bosses feel about employees and their ideas. Voice qualities—the pitch, rhythm, hoarseness, and loudness of spoken words—vary with changes in psychological arousal, emotion, and mood. They also carry social information, as when a boss speaks in angry, sarcastic, or superior tones. To the emotional brain, a biting voice hurts as much as a bite with real teeth. Neurologically, and in the same brain modules, both register as pain.

The more threatening or aggressive an animal becomes, the lower and harsher its voice turns—thus, the bigger it seems (Hopson 1980, 83). Research suggests that when two people converse, the person with the deeper, lower-frequency voice is perceived by both as having the higher social status (Schwartz 1996). According to biologist Eugene Morton, almost all mammalian sounds are blends of three basic vocalizations: growls, barks, and whines. Martha's deep voice loomed larger than most.

When the cameras were switched off, she erupted in a lava flow of barked commands and foul language (Byron 2002, 301).

In his book *Martha Stewart—Just Desserts*, Jerry Oppenheimer paints a similar picture of the ex-CEO. Not even Stewart's mother, Martha Kostyra, escaped her wrath. Stewart reportedly bellowed at, berated, and picked on her mother as she worked on assignments at her daughter's Westport, Connecticut, catering business. In describing Martha Stewart, words like "intolerance," "furious," "seething," "raging," "barking," and "acid tongue" appear throughout Oppenheimer's text. She belittled by giving off big-seeming screams, thumping gestures, and bullying barks.

Martha grew in perceived size just as animals inflate to look bigger. Puffer fish and codfish turn the widest part of their bodies toward rivals. Frogs puff up fraudulently and make deep, croaking sounds to loom larger in the pond. Lizards stiffen all four legs in aggressive high-stand displays. Cats, dogs, and other furbearers enlarge with bristling big hair. Mountain gorillas beat upon broadened chests and threaten with ear-piercing roars. Creatures take charge with bodies and gestures that connote greater size.

Through the years, Martha Stewart's stature grew "taller." That the potential for corporate malfeasance was there all along was evident in her imperial body language. On January 6, 2006, the Second U.S. Circuit Court of Appeals in Manhattan upheld Stewart's 2004 conviction.

While she was talking to me (Martha would never "chat"), I had ample time to study her face and her body language at (very) close range. She does *not* relax. I found it impossible to imagine Martha lazing in a bubble bath, or even reading a book in the shade on a beach. Martha on holiday? Impossible to envisage.

—Anne Garber, Vancouver, British Columbia, journalist (Garber 2003)

ANDREW "STEALTH" FASTOW

On January 14, 2004, Andrew S. Fastow, forty-two, pleaded guilty in a Houston federal court to two counts of wire and securities fraud for his part in the Enron accounting scandal. Dressed in a business suit, the boyish, prematurely gray Fastow showed no emotion during the proceedings. Recall from Martha Stewart's poker face that showing no emotion in court gives nonverbal testimony to guilt.

Enron, once the leading energy-trading company in the United States, filed for bankruptcy in December 2001. Thousands of Enron workers lost their jobs, stock equity, and life savings. Fastow, ex–Enron chief financial officer (CFO) and an architect of the company's spectacular nosedive, agreed to a ten-year prison sentence without parole, on condition that he cooperate with authorities on the case.

If Martha Stewart flaunted her stature to succeed in business, Andy Fastow succeeded through stealth. In his book *Anatomy of Greed*, Brian Cruver described Fastow as a quiet, low-profile executive who worked "behind the curtain" (Cruver 2002, 126–27). What Fastow did behind the curtain was use clever accounting skills to hide billions of dollars of Enron debt in "off-the-books" partnership accounts. In the process, he secretly siphoned off tens of millions of dollars for himself.

In 1997, to blend into Enron's upper echelons, Fastow hired an image consultant to advise him on clothing and ways to project an executive appearance (Murphy 2002). To look more powerful, he wore double-breasted suits with wide lapels. Some at Enron thought he looked too ostentatious, "like a gangster" (Murphy 2002). According to news accounts, Fastow was a well-groomed charmer who beamed big smiles to fit in and seemed more benign than he was (Murphy 2002). Far from benign, of course, Fastow worked undercover to relieve Enron of much of its fortune.

Like Martha Stewart, Fastow showed Jekyll-and-Hyde mood swings from "good guy" to "bad guy." The bad guy reportedly had a hair-trigger temper, publicly belittled people in meetings, and launched aggressive tirades at critics and colleagues alike. Former associates report that Fastow used a screaming, table-pounding management style and that "he loved to make people look stupid" (Zellner et al. 2002). Like Stewart's, his demeanor showed the capacity for corporate wrongdoing before he stepped into crime.

> One minute he wore his pleasant smile and his dark eyes shone. Then something would set him off. He'd twist his head, stretch his neck, and jut his chin, like a boxer warming up in the ring. The torrent of curses followed (Swartz 2003, 73).

A revealing early clue was that, unlike most CFOs, Fastow avoided dealing with market analysts outside his own Enron fiefdom. For the sake of secrecy, perhaps, Andy's posture with non-Enron analyst peers was curiously standoffish. Since his finance group was insulated, it was not subject to the same institutional controls as other company subunits. His stealthy, behind-the-curtain management style enabled him to fly largely undetected beneath corporate radar. If there were questions, he could always fall back on his winning smile. As a former high school teacher put it, Andy "used his smile as a tool" (Murphy 2002).

A second danger sign was Fastow's collection of showy properties—the large home in Southampton, the vacation homes in Galveston and Vermont, membership in the exclusive Briar Club, his Porsche 911, his wife's Mercedes-Benz, a pricey art collection, and the extravagant mansion he was building in River

Oaks (Murphy 2002). Like his costly business suits and $9,000 Franck Muller wristwatch (Anonymous 2002), Andy's properties stood out as ostentatious. "Ostentation," the nineteenth-century clergyman Edwin Chapin wrote, "is the signal flag of hypocrisy." Fastow and his wife should certainly have been wealthy, but perhaps not as wealthy as their possessions suggested. Clearly, extra cash flowed from somewhere, and suspicion turned to the CFO's corporate compensation.

In the context of a company accused of fraudulent accounting schemes, Andy's Enron paychecks seemed too big for comfort. On October 19, 2001, *The Wall Street Journal* reported that he'd received $7 million in one year's compensation from a single account known as LJM (Swartz 2003, 308). The newspaper article prompted Enron's board to investigate. At first cowed by Fastow's nasty temper, investigators eventually got him to tell how much, in total, he'd earned on his LJM account: $58.9 million (Swartz 2003, 309–10). Fastow was fired on October 24, just days after the *Journal* had raised suspicions.

A third danger sign was Fastow's bullying. As Andy became more desperate to do deals with investors to bring in revenues and bolster his leveraged accounts, he resorted to browbeating. As Mimi Swartz wrote in her book *Power Failure*, "Anyone who slowed down a deal moving toward a successful closing—an obstreperous in-house lawyer, a cautious banker, a plodding accountant—found himself a target of Fastow's anger" (Swartz 2003, 156). Like Martha Stewart, Andy bullied to seem more menacing. His increasingly malign behavior signaled that corruption was at hand.

"Fury twisted Fastow's face," Kurt Eichenwald wrote in his book *Conspiracy of Fools* (Eichenwald 2005, 134). In the incident Eichenwald described, Andy furiously glared at Enron colleague Amanda Martin and accused her of sabotaging one of his bank deals. To glare is to deliver a fierce, fixed, angry stare. In the primate world, our monkey and ape cousins stare to give threat gestures. Staring "aims" one's own personal presence, makes it feel closer, and adds a hint of looming physical contact. "If I were you," Andy threatened Amanda, "I would be very, very careful" (Eichenwald 2005, 134).

Psychologists identify bullying as one of the most stable of all human behaviors. It may begin in childhood and continue as an adult coping style. "Bullies turn into antisocial adults," Hara Marano wrote in *Psychology Today*, "and are far more likely than nonaggressive kids to commit crimes, batter their wives, abuse their children—and produce another generation of bullies" (Marano 1995). Bullies use aggressive body language to control others—by losing control of themselves. In the corporate cases of Fastow, Martha Stewart, and other top executives—including poster bad boy Ivan Boesky (see next page)—chronic anger, glaring, yelling, screaming, and table pounding correlate well with corruption.

In a January 14, 2004, Justice Department press release, Andrew Fastow was accused of having "constructed an elaborate wall of deceit—shielding the reality of Enron's failing business from the watchful eye of shareholders and the investing public." Hiding for years behind his wall of deception, Andy was virtually invisible to all but Enron insiders.

Invisibility is the nonverbal condition of being difficult or impossible to see, as in the use of camouflage, concealment, flatness, thinness, hiding, or transparency. Animals from jellyfish to human beings have devised ingenious ways to be stealthy and avoid detection.

Since jellyfish have no place to hide in the featureless ocean depths, they rely on transparency. Their clear, gelatinous bodies allow light to pass through, enabling the simple creatures to sneak up on prey while avoiding detection. Andy used transparency in the jellyfish sense—not in the human sense of being open, candid, and honest—to hide his shell-game transactions from public view. By the time people saw, Enron was already collapsing.

In the realm of big business, a human may become functionally invisible by keeping a low profile, remaining silent, and spending a great deal of time secluded behind closed doors. This Fastow did well—despite his penchant for gangster garb—until Enron's house of cards publicly imploded. When the federal government shined a light on Enron, Andrew Fastow was forced out of his corporate cocoon and was prominently featured in the news. Had the company minded his crime signals earlier, Andy might not have mattered.

IVAN BOESKY, BAD BOY

Ivan F. Boesky combined bullying and stealth to become one of the highest-paid white-collar criminals of the 1980s. He was also one of the first investigated by the U.S. Securities and Exchange Commission for investments based on information extracted from corporate insiders.

On May 18, 1986, Ivan Boesky gave a commencement address at the University of California at Berkeley. There he told business school graduates, "I think greed is healthy. You can be greedy and still feel good about yourself." Following his comment, the audience laughed and applauded (Lynn 2005).

In 2005, Boesky was listed in *Fast Company* magazine as one of the top ten "Bosses from Hell." A gaunt man who dressed in black three-piece business suits, he had prominent cheekbones, a tan face, silver-blond hair, and piercing eyes. Almost from the beginning, wrote *Den of Thieves* author James B. Stewart, Boesky "screamed at everyone regularly."

If Martha Stewart's deep voice loomed larger than most, Boesky's scream made the man's frail stature seem immense. Yelling is an active process that causes four bodily systems to tense simultaneously. The sympathetic nervous system shifts into attack mode. Heart rate and blood pressure rise. The yell's forced expiration comes as the breathing system's rib, abdominal, diaphragm, and larynx muscles contract. In explosive outbursts, muscles of the abdominal wall depress the skeletal system's lower ribs and bend the backbone and skull forward into aggressive head nods (Salmons 1995, 818–19). Like a gorilla's roar, Boesky's full-bodied scream must have filled the airspace around him.

When not screaming, yelling, or glaring, Ivan seemed mild mannered and tame. In his *New York* magazine article "Bad Boys, Bad Boys," James J. Cramer described Boesky as "almost scholarly in his demeanor." Scholarly, perhaps, but James Stewart described Boesky and his partner in crime, Michael Milken, as "the greatest criminal conspiracy the financial world has ever known."

On November 14, 1986—celebrated as "Boesky Day" on Wall Street—Ivan F. Boesky agreed to pay a court settlement of $100 million to atone for his insider-trading profits, and further agreed never again to participate in securities markets. Before stepping over the line, potential for corporate avarice was clearly reflected in his tense, confrontational body language and strident tones of voice.

JACK ABRAMOFF, GIFT GIVER

Square jawed and physically imposing—as a student, he broke the bench-press record at Beverly Hills High School—Jack A. Abramoff did not need to yell or bully his way to power. One of the most influential Washington, D.C., lobbyists of all time, until his arrest at age forty-six on indictment in Los Angeles on August 11, 2005, Abramoff used his hereditary stature to win friends and influence people.

As a child at Beverly Hills Elementary School, Abramoff reportedly tried to buy his way to student-body president by giving young voters free hot dogs (Taibbi 2006). Gift giving on a grander scale was to become his modus operandi later in life. Called "influence peddling," the giving of gifts—vacation trips, tickets to football games, free meals at his restaurant, and cash—brought others nearer to the man's side. Unlike in bullying, there were no hard feelings. Those whom Jack gifted were grateful.

Anthropologists study gift giving as a nonverbal means of exchange. Gifts themselves lack the faculty of speech but communicate essential messages and meanings apart from words. Since the 1925 publication of Marcel Mauss's classic work, *The Gift*, ethnologists have recognized the immense power of giving in human relationships. Mauss taught that gifts are never free. Anthropologists today agree that when accepted, gifts incur strong obligations. Accepting a gift carries an implicit obligation to reciprocate in kind.

On March 31, 2006, Tony Rudy pleaded guilty to conspiracy charges in U.S. District Court in Washington, D.C. According to court papers, Rudy, a former staff member for U.S. representative Tom DeLay of Texas, helped Abramoff stop legislation opposed by one of his clients, the Commonwealth of Northern Marianas Islands (CNMI). The CNMI paid Abramoff $7.17 million in lobbying fees, and Abramoff used part of the money to compensate Capitol Hill insider Rudy with "free trips, sporting tickets, meals and golf games and $86,000 [given] to a consulting firm he set up [that] was run by his wife" (Seidman 2006).

Like the Trobriand Islands' "Kula Ring," in which Solomon Sea trading partners exchange highly valued shell ornaments from island to island, the Abramoff gift kept on giving. According to court papers, Rudy used Abramoff funds to provide "things of value" to Representative Bob Ney (R-Ohio) in the form of partial payment for a golfing trip to Scotland. Ney then agreed, in March 2001, to support legislation favorable to Abramoff's CNMI client (Seidman 2006). As in the Trobriand Islands, gifts that go around come around.

Along with gifting, Abramoff used the nonverbal ploy of showing. To see a physical object or commodity is more convincing than merely to hear about it in words. Often skeptical about verbal statements we hear, we naively trust what our eyes can see. Jack Abramoff's SunCruz deal is a case in point.

On March 29, 2006, Abramoff was sentenced in a Florida federal court to five years and ten months in prison for conspiracy and wire fraud in the purchase of SunCruz Casinos in the year 2000 (Dahlburg 2006). Before sentencing, Abramoff sat in silence in the courtroom. His eyes were closed. Later, outside, he did not answer reporters' questions. Instead of wearing his trademark gangster hat, characterized by *Rolling Stone* magazine as a "Boris Badenov fedora," Abramoff wore a friendlier, tan-colored baseball cap, perhaps as a sign intended to show that he'd changed his ways.

Six years before the sentencing, Jack Abramoff and his partner, Adam Kidan, had taken over SunCruz Casinos, a firm that operated a fleet of gambling boats from seaports in Florida. They bought SunCruz from Konstantinos "Gus" Boulis, founder of the Miami Subs sandwich chain (Grimaldi 2005). To buy the business, Abramoff and Kidan borrowed money from individuals to display as "flash funds," to show potential lenders they had enough money to purchase the firm. Since we trust our own eyes, "seeing is believing."

To borrow from financial institutions, the partners faked their wealth with paper. In the cargo cults of Papua New Guinea, a culture area that includes the Trobriand Islands, "magical" pieces of paper were circulated by natives who had watched New Guinea–based U.S. soldiers circulate invoices for cargo received at their ports and airbases during World War II. The Stone Age natives saw paperwork as a magical means to acquire the soldiers' bountiful supply of canned goods, radios, chocolate bars, and other wondrous cargo. Abramoff's own magical papers showed that $23 million—funds the partners themselves committed toward acquiring SunCruz—had been transferred to their corporate account for the sale. The wire transfer itself, however, "was counterfeit," said R. Alexander Acosta, the U.S. attorney in Miami. Nonetheless, seeing is believing had worked twice.

If deceptive flash funds and bogus pieces of paper rang "true" without sounding an alarm, what happened next overflowed with transparent crime signals. After Abramoff and Kidan bought SunCruz, Gus Boulis remained a partner in the deal. Yet Boulis was unhappy, and accused Kidan of having links to organized crime. Boulis and Kidan reportedly came to blows at a business meeting, and according to the *The Washington Post*, "Immediately after the fight, Abramoff agreed with Kidan in e-mails that Boulis should be removed from SunCruz" (Grimaldi 2005).

On February 6, 2001, Konstantinos Boulis was killed in his car by a drive-by shooter, who was never identified, and two of the three men arrested in connection with the ambush slaying of Boulis had been previously hired as consultants by Kidan. Neither of the two remaining SunCruz partners was charged with the crime. What began for Jack Abramoff with gifts—hot dogs, meals, golf games, and cash—ended with fists, bullets, indictments, and guilty pleas. That he would step over the line into white-collar crime was evident, nonverbally, in the extravagant gifts he gave. As French anthropologist Marcel Mauss taught more than eighty years ago, gifts are almost never free.

White-collar criminals are among the most secretive of lawbreakers. They are not often pictured on the glossy pages of stockholder reports. To find these elusive offenders, we must watch their actions, read their body language, and listen to their tones of voice. Since tiny muscles of the voice box are linked to emotionally sensitive, special visceral nerves, the manner in which they speak can be as telling as their words—or more so. An imperious voice tone correlates well with the supposition that one stands above the law.

To catch a white-collar thief in action, watch for signs suggesting that all is not well in the executive suite:

- Screaming, yelling, and bullying in the office
- Belittling speech tones
- Stealthy, secretive demeanor
- A CEO's pouting, frowning, or chronically clenched jaw
- A CFO's glare that could kill
- Gratuitous ostentation in clothing, possessions, and lifestyle
- The offer of "free" gifts

You have seen how stature, stealth, bullying, and gift giving are instrumental to the commission of white-collar crimes. In the next chapter, you will learn to decode the nonverbal language of those who take, share, and traffic in drugs.

10

THE SYMBOLS OF AN ADDICTION

In brightest day, in darkest night, no evil shall escape my
sight, for I am the Shadow Wolf.

—Motto of the Shadow Wolves, Native American
trackers who stalk drug smugglers

"CARL HAD ALWAYS assured me that he wasn't using alcohol or
drugs," his mother, Misty Fetko, wrote of her oldest son. In her
article on the Web site of the Partnership for a Drug-Free America, she added, "I knew he was a good kid and I believed him."
The boy had just graduated from high school and was preparing
to leave in two days for the Memphis College of Art.

Every mother wants to believe her child's words, but earlier
Fetko had found likely signs of drug abuse. The English word
"sign" comes from Latin *signum*, "identifying mark." "Sign" is
the general term for any physical object, movement, or quality
that communicates or carries information. In philosophy, as de-
fined by Charles S. Peirce, "a sign stands for something else"
(Flew 1979, 327).

Misty Fetko had found signs of marijuana in her son's bedroom during his junior year in high school, and empty bottles of cough syrup in their basement after a summer night's sleepover with friends (Fetko 2006). These signs plainly stood for something else, and the something was drug use. An Ohio registered nurse who worked in a hospital emergency room, Fetko was alert to drug symptoms, and vigilant about keeping narcotics out of her home. The marijuana was a clear "indexical" sign of usage, just as footprints are indexical signs of the feet that leave them. The meaning of empty cough-syrup bottles, however, was less transparent. For starters, why were there more than one? Misty was unaware that, like her own son, high school kids had begun using cold and cough medicines to get high. This was 2003, before "Robotripping"—named for the cough medicine Robitussin—had evolved into the teen drug fashion it was to become.

On the night of July 15, 2003, Misty and Carl chatted about his upcoming journey from home in Ohio to school in Memphis, Tennessee. He smiled, hugged his mother, and said, "Goodnight, Mom. Love you" (Fetko 2006).

The next morning, July 16, Misty Fetko found Carl dead in his bedroom from a drug overdose that had lethally arrested his breathing sometime in the night. She tried CPR to revive him but tragically failed. He had died with a combination of three drugs in his body: marijuana; fentanyl, a prescription narcotic pain reliever; and dextromethorphan, or DXM, the hallucinatory cough suppressant used in over-the-counter cold remedies.

In her effort to keep Carl drug free, Misty had watched for typical, textbook signs such as hash pipes, bongs, and cigarette papers. "But there were no needles, no powders, no smells, no large amounts of money being spent," she wrote (Fetko 2006). Yes, there was the specter of marijuana, but Misty didn't consider cannabis a dangerous drug like heroin or meth. She did not know until after her son died that kids were drinking up to four bottles a day of cough syrup—a potentially deadly dosage—to dissociate from reality.

On behalf of her son, Misty Fetko became a national spokeswoman for the Partnership for a Drug-Free America. From her own and Carl's terrible experience, we know more about drug signs today. His use of marijuana was a sign of experimentation, which in teenagers is an active, ongoing process that tends to ratchet upward rather than wane. Moreover, young people today eagerly share information on the Internet about new drugs and novel narcotic blends. There is intense peer pressure to dare, take risks, and step ahead of friends in drug abuse. Carl himself kept a computer journal of the drug experiments he'd tried. To keep up with current drug signs, signals, and cues, parents must enter the child's electronic world to see inside their children's minds.

"Be involved in your kids' lives," Fetko advises, "and talk to them regularly about the dangers of drugs. Don't be afraid of questioning them. Don't be afraid of being a pest."

DRUG SIGNALS

The drug world teems with crime signals throughout its tangled distribution web. Clues left by smugglers, couriers, dealers, and users are as varied as any unearthed by the master detective Sherlock Holmes. Holmes could unlock a case by detecting traces of disinfectant left on a glove, or by nebulous shoe marks imprinted in sand. In Holmes's world, the most trivial crime signal could unlock the most consequential case.

Along the U.S.-Mexican border today, Shadow Wolves read footprints to detect drug smugglers who move marijuana under cover of darkness into the desert Southwest. Shadow Wolves are Native Americans from the Navaho, Tohono O'odham, and other Indian tribes who are special agents of the U.S. Department of Homeland Security. They are the best trackers in the world. The sour smell of body odor, the sight of burlap fibers dangling from a strand of barbed wire, or the presence of freshly broken twigs on the desert sand could be clues of a drug smuggler's nocturnal presence.

Shadow Wolves call their interdiction work "cutting for sign." Sign is the physical, tangible, gritty evidence they use to track down secretive bands of men carrying burlap bundles of illegal drugs en route to sale in U.S. neighborhoods. Before making a capture, Shadow Wolves may tail a smuggler band for two to three days across the Arizona desert.

Despite their best efforts, huge quantities of drugs get through for sale on the street. From Arizona highways, the next stop in the covert distribution chain is the local neighborhood. A typical locale was once the 700 block of North Monticello Avenue in Chicago, Illinois. (Vigilant neighbors shut down the operation a few years ago.) According to the commander of Chicago's Eleventh Police District, "A lot of times, drug dealers will look for areas that are unkempt," and Monticello Avenue fit the profile (Mister 2003). At a vacant lot across from an elementary school, loitering dealers quietly sold to a "steady flow" of buyers. According to one resident, "It looked like people were buying groceries" (Mister 2003).

In case the Chicago police came calling, drug dealers were smart enough not to hold contraband themselves. Instead, they hid drugs in secret locations. When customers paid, dealers would gesture toward the stash. Observant officers who knew where to look for clues found drugs squirreled away in trees, between lawns and sidewalks, concealed in woodpiles, and hidden behind tires, under cars, and even in gas tanks. From the lowly jellyfish to human beings, animals have devised ingenious ways to avoid detection, and drug dealers are no exception.

Buyers are no less secretive. Needle users cover injection marks with long sleeves, even in hot weather. Marijuana smokers conceal reddened eyes with sunglasses, even indoors, and with eyedrops. Cocaine users make frequent trips to vacant rooms, storage areas, and basements for no obvious reason. Gratuitous coming and going can be a sign that something illegal is going on.

JUST HIKING . . . TO CANADA

On March 11, 2006, U.S. Customs and Border Protection agents captured $3.1 million in cocaine in a rural area near Oroville, Washington (Ferrer 2006). Suspicions were aroused when they saw three men with backpacks walking north toward the Canadian border. The "hike" in this locality seemed unusual. When agents approached to question the men, the suspects fled. As courts now interpret the Fourth Amendment to the U.S. Constitution, physical flight from officers is probable cause for detention. Agents recovered the drugs after the men dropped their packs and ran away. Despite their escape, the men's anomalous movements led to one of the biggest drug seizures in eastern Washington history.

At a body-language seminar I gave in Beaumont, Texas, for the Road Warrior Interdiction Network (RWIN), an organization of highway narcotics interdiction officers from across the United States and Canada, police officers described a telltale guilty sign suspects display when stopped on suspicion of drug transport: a suspect exits his vehicle and—before any discussion with officers—puts his hands behind his back in anticipation of being cuffed. For officers, the hands-behind-back sign is a gratuitous indication of guilt. The suspect inadvertently tips police that he's carrying illegal drugs.

Other suspicious signs, according to Beaumont Police Department narcotics interdiction officer Gerald P. LaChance, include "religious bumper stickers, Bibles on the dash, religious music playing, 'I Support My Local Police' stickers, and any other items that the violator may use to try to get officers to believe he's a good person" (LaChance 2005).

Law enforcement benefits, as well, from eye-catching drug paraphernalia. Colorful bongs, roach clips, miniature spoons, and fancy pipes make consuming illicit drugs highly visible. Ornate designs are governed by a principle of what I call "nonverbal independence." Like the aroma of blossoms, herbs, and medicinal plants, ornamentation in paraphernalia design evolved apart from structural needs for functionality and durability. A bong's or drug pipe's decorations are purely for show. Thanks to nonverbal independence, drug paraphernalia have a lot to "say." And, clearly, police are listening.

WHAT'S THE MATTER WITH GOODEN?

Drug symptoms often include noticeable losses in physical skills, as was classically the case for baseball superstar Dwight Gooden. A pitcher celebrated for his ability to strike out batters, Gooden won the National League's Cy Young Award in 1985 after winning its Rookie of the Year Award in 1984, and played as an All-Star in 1984, 1986, and 1988.

On March 14, 2006, Gooden was arrested for failing a drug test. On March 23, he admitted in a Tampa courtroom to using cocaine. On April 5, 2006, Dwight Gooden, forty-one, was sentenced to a year and a day in a Florida state prison for violating his probation by using the white, crystalline alkaloid.

Drug use showed not only in Gooden's demeanor, but also in his pitching. After 1985, he never again achieved the stellar domination he'd once had as baseball's strikeout king. Sportswriters around the world had begun to ask, "What's wrong with Gooden?" Most likely answer: cocaine.

BODY LANGUAGE OF METH

Methamphetamine—"meth"—is currently the fastest-growing competitor for street sales with more conventional products like powder cocaine, crack cocaine, marijuana, and heroin. Meth is the most addictive of all street drugs.

Trying meth for the first time is virtually to become addicted. "I loved it," a first-time user exclaimed. "I felt so energetic, skinny, pretty." Of all drugs, meth has the most dramatic effect on an abuser's demeanor, body language, skin, hair, and teeth. Meth users may not sleep for days; may look freakishly disheveled; and may show anxious, writhing hand movements, open sores on their bodies, patches of hair picked away, and visibly decaying teeth.

From hundreds of anonymous personal stories made public on the Internet by KCI—"the Anti-Meth Site" (www.kci.org)—a revealing portrait of meth users emerges:

- *A "friend" entices a friend to partake.* "We sat on her bed and she lit it for me." "I was sitting at my desk at work crying when a so-called friend came over. She told me she had something that would help." "He said he felt incredible, he seemed so happy and excited and awake. He wanted me to try it too."
- *Bodily symptoms soon appear.* "I couldn't stop clenching my jaw." "My hands shake all the time." "I lost 50 pounds in two or three months." "I

could see my hipbones and my thighbones through my legs. All of my ribs showed." "Corey looked like a skeleton of his former handsome self." "In front of the mirror, I picked at my face and scraped away worms that were never really there." "My face and body were covered in sores and cysts from the endless picking." "I used to be pretty; my teeth are falling out." "I am 31 years old and saving money for dentures."

· *Others notice.* "My friends said I wasn't blinking, I was just staring straight through them." "He'd known something was wrong with me, but had no idea the degree of what I'd done." "My 3 year old is always asking me what's wrong and if I am ok."

Methamphetamine is easily manufactured in small home-based labs from commercially available products. Watch your neighborhood for such warning signs as: (1) strong odors of acetone, ammonia, and ether; (2) unusual quantities of clear glass containers; (3) reclusive neighbors who rarely notice you—and never greet you; (4) antifreeze containers, coffee filters stained red, drain cleaner; and (5) residential windows blacked out with blankets, plywood, or aluminum foil.

DECEPTION RUNS RAMPANT

Recall from chapter 1 that lawbreakers lie to cover up their offenses. Drug users lie for another reason, as well: to feed their addiction. Nothing is more important than obtaining more drugs. As thirty-year-old "George," a member of Narcotics Anonymous, explained in his personal narrative: "Now it was conning, ripping people off and doing whatever was necessary to get narcotics" (Anonymous 1988, 184).

George used codeine, heroin, marijuana, methadone, methamphetamine, and prescription drugs. At one point he had sores in his mouth, yellow skin, and hallucinations. Since his vision didn't focus at night, he stayed indoors. As George himself admitted, "I had become a garbage can for drugs" (Anonymous 1988, 185). Toward the end of his addiction, he switched from street drugs to prescription drugs obtained from doctors. Like many addicts, George was a skillful liar when it came to conning drugs from medical professionals.

In a second Narcotics Anonymous confession, "Jo," a housewife, admitted she'd learned from a hospital stay that she could manipulate symptoms to acquire drugs. "My life became one of appointments to doctors' offices, lies to them and to myself, prescriptions and trips to the hospital" (Anonymous 1988, 190). She went through unnecessary surgeries purely for the sake of using drugs. Fortunately, through Narcotics Anonymous, both George and Jo overcame their addiction to narcotics—and to lying to doctors.

NEEDLE DECEPTION

"The needle slowly became my friend, lover and my reason for living," a young woman wrote in her Narcotics Anonymous story (Anonymous 1988, 171). Eventually, when telltale sores showed on her body— "from my head to my toes"—her daughter and parents noticed. To cover up the all-too-visible evidence of drug abuse, she told them her sores were just boils. Deception is the currency of addiction, and her sores prompted excuses.

Another confession is from a doctor himself, a successful surgeon who became an addict. He admitted that to ease the pain of living, he gradually "crossed the magical line" between occasional user and addict. "I lied to cover up my habit," he wrote, "and yet my wife always knew" (Anonymous 1988, 201). The daily signals he gave were clear. He took drugs at the end of each workday, arrived home in a semistupor, quickly ate dinner, and went to bed early. Reading between the lines, she knew something was wrong. His something was needles and pills.

At work, sensing from the addict's physical and emotional condition that something was wrong, colleagues insisted that he seek help. In the initial consultation, as he started to explain the drug problem, his counselor "held up his hand as if to say stop. 'You're addicted'" (Anonymous 1988, 202). After a stay in drug rehabilitation, the surgeon joined Narcotics Anonymous and, like George and Jo, overcame his addiction to narcotics—and to lying to himself.

NONVERBAL DELIGHT

Pleasure's a sin, and sometimes sin's a pleasure.

—BYRON, *Don Juan*, canto 1

Few activities in the crime world are as addictive as doing drugs. Reasons for narco-passion lie in an ancient part of the brain called the pleasure pathway. The five-hundred-million-year-old pleasure pathway begins in the middle of the brain and extends to an addiction center at the front of the brain called the nucleus accumbens. The nucleus accumbens is centrally located at the intersection of reptilian basal ganglia, where many body movements are begun and controlled, and the mammalian brain's limbic system, where emotion resides.

Since it originated hundreds of millions of years before the advent of speech, I call the pleasure pathway a "nonverbal" part of the brain. People were motivated by pleasure aeons before they were motivated by words.

Drugs like cocaine and meth instantly and dramatically stimulate the pleasure pathway. Sex arouses the pathway as well. Brain researchers have learned that pleasure is remarkably the same whether initiated by drugs, sex, or rock and roll. Additionally, we find pleasure in discovery, ideation, and knowledge. As cosmologist Stephen Hawking put it, "There's nothing like the Eureka moment, of discovering something that no one knew before. I won't compare it to sex, but it lasts longer."

The allure of drugs is that they provide quick, easy, and dramatic entry to the pleasure pathway. Socrates, Plato, Freud, and Picasso reportedly used mind-altering drugs. The fictional detective Sherlock Holmes, as well, injected cocaine three times daily in *The Sign of Four*. At the time, drugs were not illegal. The problem today is that narcotics are too poweful, too available, and too addicting. Drugs like meth quickly exhaust the pleasure pathway, the body, the mind, and ultimately, the soul. And today's drugs are illegal.

SIGN OF THE TIMES: JESÚS MALVERDE

From Sinaloa, Mexico, to Fresno, California, shrines have been set up to honor "the patron saint of drug traffickers," Jesús Malverde. Seeing the likeness of Malverde's dark hair and iconic black mustache in someone's home is a good sign that drug traffickers live there. As Sergeant Alex Flores of the Fresno Police Department's major narcotics unit said, "It just kind of lets us know this person is into the [drug] business beyond the superficial" (Eberly 2005).

Drug dealers display porcelain statues of the Robin Hood–like Mexican folk hero to protect themselves from capture by police. Police in Bakersfield, California, estimate that up to 80 percent of Mexican nationals involved in the drug trade display Malverde symbolism on personal items.

Placed in a washroom, bedroom, or living room corner or closet, Malverde shrines are kept meticulously clean and are decorated with fresh flowers and lit candles. When police ask drug dealers about the statues, "We get a lot of varied responses," Sergeant Flores reports. "I'd say the biggest response is we get a smile and a nod" (Eberly 2005).

This classic "walking-corpse" caricature of drug users first appeared in 1838 in an article from the *Boston Medical and Surgical Journal* (Anonymous 1838):

The habitual opium eater is instantly recognized by his appearance. A total attenuation of body, a withered, yellow countenance, a lame gait, a bending of the spine, frequently to such a degree as to assume a circular form, and glossy, deep-sunken eyes, betray him at first glance.

Using it today, you would miss literally millions of users who abuse drugs yet manage to escape notice and blend into normal family, school, and workplace routines. To detect present-day drug abusers, watch for the following signs:

· dilated pupils (methamphetamine, cocaine)
· constricted pupils (codeine, heroin, methadone, morphine, opium)
· rapid eye movements (ecstasy)
· inflammation and redness in whites of eyes (marijuana)
· frequent lip licking (methamphetamine, cocaine)
· acute runny nose (cocaine)
· itchy skin (methamphetamine)
· delusions of parasites, insects, or worms on the skin (methamphetamine)
· absent facial expressions (codeine, heroin, methadone, morphine, opium)
· excessively animated facial expressions (methamphetamine, cocaine)
· rapid weight loss (methamphetamine)
· jaw clenching, muscle tension (ecstasy, methamphetamine, cocaine)

- excessive bodily activity or movement (methamphetamine, cocaine)
- anxiety, nervousness (methamphetamine)
- picking at skin, pulling out hair (methamphetamine)
- slow writhing or jerky, flailing hand movements (methamphetamine)
- tremors (alcoholism, methamphetamine)
- lethargy, flat behavioral affect (codeine, heroin, methadone, morphine, opium)
- slurred speech (alcohol, codeine, heroin, methadone, morphine, opium)
- loud group laughter (marijuana)
- profuse sweating (ecstasy, methamphetamine)
- facial flushing or paleness (assorted narcotics)
- facial acne, bodily sores (methamphetamine)
- sudden outbursts of anger (methamphetamine)
- abrupt changes in personal cleanliness and grooming (all, with heavy use)
- slowed driving (alcohol, marijuana)
- droopy eyelids (cough syrup—dextromethorphan)

In the next and final chapter, you will learn to decipher the body language of thieves. Thieves are the most generic of all criminals. From con men to pedophiles, from murderers to stalkers to terrorists, all criminals take something from us bodily, mentally, or spiritually. Staying alert to crime signals will safeguard against those who would rip you off.

11

TO CATCH A THIEF

In more severe forms, any visual target will elicit manual reaching
followed by tight grasping.

—M. MARSEL MESULAM,
on the grasping reflex

IN ITS MOST basic sense, theft is the physical act of taking something illegally by means of grasping. A thief is one who steals another's property—usually by stealth rather than force—employing
the hands to take ownership. To surreptitiously pinch, cop, hook,
lift, swipe, palm, or rip off suggests seizing with the terminal end
organs below the forearms, the fingers and hands.

In May 2006, rampant theft was reported in several wealthy
oceanfront communities along South Africa's Cape Peninsula
near the city of Cape Town. Grasping hands had reached into
pantries, refrigerators, and fruit bowls in an unchecked crime
wave of thievery (Ferreira 2006).

One resident of the Cape Peninsula district watched as a thief
"just flew through the burglar bars and into the house" in search
of items to steal (Ferreira 2006). Earlier, the same culprit was

seen sauntering into a neighbor's home, where he opened the re-frigerator, removed eggs, and scattered them on the floor (Fer-reira 2006). Longtime area residents said the thieves had lived in harmony with neighbors for decades, until tourists began giving free handouts. Free food apparently prompted the burglars to help themselves.

Cape Peninsula's grasping hands, you probably guessed, be-long not to people but to monkeys: the area's resident baboons. Theft as human beings know it has deep roots in animal psychol-ogy. In fact, our earliest ancestors likely stole before they could speak.

Theft is common among primates today. In a study of wild chimpanzees living in Uganda's Kibale National Park, primatolo-gists John Mitani and David Watts observed 113 instances of males sharing meat—and 26 instances of males stealing meat from each other (Mitani and Watts 1999). "Meat theft," they wrote, "occurred quickly and either high in the trees or as animals rushed rapidly along the ground" (Mitani and Watts 1999, 444).

On November 6, 2002, Mustapha Riat of London, England, awoke to the sound of scratching and saw a chimpanzee's hairy arm reach through his bedroom window and grab his cell phone (O'Neill 2002). Police officers who responded to the theft said they'd just come from another chimp burglary in the neighbor-hood, in which a watch had been taken from Ms. Gina Davidson's mantel.

In New Delhi, India, rhesus monkeys routinely break into homes and offices to steal food, lunch boxes, and random valu-ables such as whiskey, cell phones, mail, and even top secret doc-uments. In the 1995 movie *Dunston Checks In*, an orangutan is trained as a jewel thief to steal from swanky hotels. A year earlier, in the 1994 film *Monkey Trouble*, the jewel thief is a craftily trained capuchin monkey. In Africa, England, India, and Hollywood, the grasping digits of monkeys and apes open a window into the primate's basically purloining soul.

Theft is rooted in our own species' innate grasping reflex. On a daily basis, we are tempted by objects displayed in shop windows and on supermarket shelves. Thanks to the grasping reflex, we have a strong desire to pick up, handle, and hold material objects, especially items of elegant design such as gold coins, platinum rings, and diamond bracelets. For some, the grasping urge may be too powerful to resist.

Neurologist Marsel Mesulam explains that for people with severe forms of the grasping reflex, objects become magnetic, and "any visual target will elicit manual reaching followed by tight grasping" (Mesulam 1992, 696). I call our fascination with material things "object fancy." Manufactured products call to us nonverbally through exhibited "gestures." Design features—the sheen, shape, and smoothness of a bracelet or gold ring—send compelling messages that capture our attention, interest, and fancy.

Forever beckoning from TV commercials and magazine ads, products gesture until we answer their call. When I was nine, I received a powerful call from a cache of colorless artificial gems known as rhinestones. I was mesmerized by the sparkle as they lay scattered on a tabletop in my neighbor's sewing room. I knew the gems belonged to Richard's mom, but so strong was my urge to grasp them that I went back, when no one was home, and seized the gleaming stones in my palms.

So strong was my urge to grasp them that I went back, when no one was home, and seized the gleaming stones in my palms.

Everyone remembers that peculiar childhood moment when the urge to steal something precious gave way to material theft. I recall my own rhinestone caper as intensely thrilling. There was an adrenal flash of excitement in the darkened sewing room as, with pounding heart and trembling hands, I realized the gems were "mine." I dreamed of a future career as a jewel thief. Of course, when Mother saw my precious treasure trove, the jig was up. With bowed head and downcast eyes, I returned the rhinestones and tearfully apologized. Prospects for a Pink Panther career were as empty as my open palms.

I could have been a master jewel thief like William Mason. Mason began his career in the 1960s and stole for thirty years from such notables as Truman Capote, Phyllis Diller, Robert Goulet, Armand Hammer, and Bob Hope (Mason 2003). Described as "shadowy, elusive, and intensely private," he single-handedly stole more than $35 million worth of fabulous jewelry.

Yet while charming his way into high society to take from the rich and famous, Mason maintained a double life as an outwardly ordinary real estate investor and family man. Like many thieves, he was a study in plainness. Unlike murderers, who direct their violence at another; swindlers, who need people to fool; and gang members, who seek out a group to belong to, thieves are happiest when no one's around. A compulsion for secrecy makes a thief's crime signals harder to see. Like the elusive "hidden animals" studied by cryptozoologists, thieves hide their existence to remain unseen.

In William Mason's case, his own physical presence while casing hotels, observing workday routines, and planning escape routes might have seemed suspicious had he not dressed as an ordinary man. To remain undetected, neither his clothing nor his persona stood out. Unlike a gang member, who needs to be seen, Mason was both there and not there at the same time.

WITHOUT RAISING EYEBROWS

By his own admission, George N. Feder of Florida stole a small fortune's worth of jewelry over a ten-year period. "I walked into high-rise, luxury condominiums with nothing but a smile, nice clothes and a couple of lock-picking tools and walked out with diamonds, emeralds, sapphires, rubies, gold and other special items," he wrote in "Confessions of an Ex–Jewel Thief" (Feder 2001).

George liked robbing condominiums because their owners felt "safe" inside, with locked gates, security systems, and supposedly watchful doormen. Since condo security was more relaxed during daylight hours, that's when he robbed, often by picking a lock on a side-entry door.

As a teenager, George Feder studied lock picking from an expert, a fellow jewel thief from his old neighborhood in New York. Feder learned how to place his index finger on the pick to feel inside the lock as its tiny pins pushed up. "It's all in the feel," his teacher explained.

In public, Feder was something of a showman. He carried monogrammed lock picks, wore a four-carat diamond ring, and drove a yellow Cadillac El Dorado convertible. He relished the glamour of being a jewel thief. "I was fascinated by jewelry, the look of it, the feel of it," Feder confessed (Feder 2001). Like William Mason, George Feder made sure to fit in on the job and not stand out while robbing. He wore tennis shoes and polo shirts, gripped a tennis racket, and carried a tennis bag to stash jewels in so he could pass by people, as he put it, "without raising eyebrows."

Feder loved being a thief. He reported feeling most alive in dangerous situations that kindled the "hot rush of adrenaline" (Feder 2001). As a bonus, stealing jewels made him feel like someone special.

Feder preferred robbing the most expensive top-floor units, corner apartments, and penthouse suites. Experience taught him that these housed the fanciest, costliest jewels. Before entering a building, he drove by neighboring condos to check for addresses. An address was always handy to have in case someone stopped him in a hallway.

"I'm looking for John Smith in 906," he might say.

"There's no Smith in that apartment," a resident might answer.

"Oh, is this 6641 Wakefield Drive?"

"No, it's 6631."

"Oops, my mistake." Feder would then take an elevator down to a lower floor to resume his illegal grasping. "I had to be a great actor," he wrote in his memoir (Feder 2001).

Feder noted that even the most expensive condominiums had rather dark hallways, which made facial recognition from a distance that much harder. As he padded down a condo hall, George searched for signs telling him which units to avoid and which to rob. Since doors magnify sounds, he had little difficulty hearing if occupants were home. On a hot Florida day, not hearing an air conditioner meant residents were probably out. Hearing a TV discouraged him from entering, as did the smell of cigarette smoke and the aroma of freshly cooked food.

After picking a lock to enter the chosen condo, Feder would gingerly search for valuables. He knew the best places to look, like the ever promising lingerie drawer. When the situation got tough, his heart skipped a beat, and he felt "tiny beads of sweat" on his forehead—but he wrote that his hands "remained steady" (Feder 2001).

In 1977, George Feder, master jewel thief, was finally apprehended by the FBI. Feder spent nine years in maximum-security prisons. Afterward, he reformed and became a crime-prevention consultant. Feder even designed a virtually pickproof door lock known as the "Revolution." Before his capture, George Feder's body language and demeanor—his ability to mimic the appearance of those he robbed; to convincingly act as if he were just in the "wrong" building; to smile as if all were right with the world; and, in times of stress, to keep steady hands—enabled him to rob with impunity for ten years without raising an eyebrow.

A SHIFTY LOOK IN HIS EYES

The reason George Feder stole, he wrote, was because "it made me somebody" (Feder 2001). However, life is less rewarding for ordinary robbers, who participate in the three most common types of thievery—commercial (e.g., banks and convenience stores), street theft, and residential burglary.

"I am a thief," Lowell Johnson wrote in his article "Confessions of a Convicted Vending Burglar."

"You have probably seen 2 million people who look just like me," Johnson wrote, "and never gave them a second glance" (Johnson 2005). His claim of looking "just like you and me" is commonly found in the true-crime confessionals of thieves. Johnson accuses us of having preconceptions about what the typical thief looks like: "Unkempt hair. Ratty clothes. A shifty look in his eyes" (Johnson 2005). Not true, Johnson writes: "I don't look like that."

Computer professional Lowell Johnson began his career as a thief to support an addiction to crack cocaine. His specialty was vending machines, which he burglarized after learning on the Internet how to pick locks. Johnson's first heist was from a soda machine located out of easy view in a government building's restroom. First he watched the traffic flow in and out of the restroom, and then he casually entered and picked the machine's lock in thirty seconds. His heart was racing, he recalled, as he grabbed $100 from the machine and walked out of the room.

"I then proceeded to leave the area," Johnson wrote, "watching carefully for anyone paying attention to me" (Johnson 2005). In accord with the dictum that criminals must return to the scene of the crime, he revisited the same restroom half an hour later and stole $200 from a candy machine.

Before long, Johnson's weekly routine became as regular as that of a parcel-post deliveryman. But instead of delivering, he picked locks and grabbed currency from bill holders (coins were too noisy). Johnson's physical movements through space and time soon became predictable. He would drive from town to town on the interstate, stop at a tourist information center, and ask for directions to "hospitals, colleges, hotels, and any other large public areas such as malls, bowling alleys and zoos" (Johnson 2005).

Other people, Johnson learned, were as predictable in their physical movements as he was in his. In hotels, guests were least likely to visit vending machines in the afternoon. In hospitals, the best time to rob was 8:00 p.m., and in colleges the right time was around 10:00 at night. Early morning between 6:00 and 7:00 was also mostly free of foot traffic around vending machines in colleges and hospitals.

Though he preferred privacy, Johnson learned how to act when people saw him stealing. "As long as I act like I am supposed to be there," he wrote, "most employees will not question it" (Johnson 2005). After the initial thirty- to sixty-second lock pick, he could make return visits with a preset burglar tool. Anyone who saw him then would think Johnson was a technician using an authorized key.

Unlike jewel thievery, in which hands grasp thousands of dollars in merchandise at a time, vending-machine thieves rely on volume. Since the chance of getting caught rises in direct proportion to the number of thefts, Lowell Johnson was bound to be caught—sooner rather than later—with his hands in the cookie jar. In fact, toward the end he was caught red-handed several times. Once a lounge employee saw him "poking" at a machine and called police (Johnson 2005). Johnson spent twenty days in jail for the incident. For a subsequent theft, he received thirty months in prison.

Lowell Johnson—actually the convicted burglar's pseudonym—enjoyed his work. The hours were short, and his gross pay, measured in hundreds of thousands of dollars, was generous. Since machines never fought back, the work was relatively safe. Moreover, taking from a machine spared Johnson the guilt of having to look into the emotional eyes of human victims.

GENTLEMEN BANDITS

In the media, mild-mannered, neatly dressed, soft-spoken thieves are called "gentlemen bandits." Though well armed, well-behaved bank robbers are pictured, like Robin Hood, as having hearts of gold.

Born in Transylvania, former ice-hockey player Attila Ambrus was a Hungarian bank robber known for drinking a shot of whiskey before each of his twenty-eight armed robberies, and for his gentlemanly gesture of giving flowers to the female tellers he'd robbed (Lebor 1999). Celebrated in Hungary as "the Whiskey Robber," Ambrus escaped from bank robberies in taxicabs or by bravely swimming away in the Danube. His reported take from bank heists was 142 million forints—almost $600,000. Ambrus finally confessed to his crimes and was put in a high-security prison. In July 1999, the gentleman bandit escaped down a rope of tied bedsheets.

More recently, in April 2006, the FBI asked for help in identifying a so-called gentleman bandit who robbed as many as six banks in the Chicago area (Anonymous 2006a). He was described as a tall, clean-cut, well-dressed black male in his thirties or forties who behaved politely. Though an armed robber, the suspect would apologize to bank employees, saying "times are tough."

Such is the romance of polite purloiners that a number of gentleman-bandit movies have appeared in cinema and on TV. In the 1968 cult movie *The Thomas Crown Affair*, Steve McQueen plays a rich, gentlemanly thief who races dune buggies, plays chess, and charms a beautiful insurance investigator (played by Faye Dunaway). A 2002 B movie called *The Gentleman Bandit* features a well-dressed, handsome man with a Band-Aid over his nose who robs several banks in Beverly Hills. In the crime world, a polite demeanor does not go unnoticed.

BARBARIANS ON THE STREET

Street theft is the most common brand of thievery in the U.S. today, accounting for half of all reported theft cases. Street thieves confront victims personally, directly, often face-to-face. They may speak, gesture, and make eye contact. Since some victims fight back, street thieves must always be prepared to use physical force. These offenders are aggressive, predatory, and always dangerous.

Street robbers tend to behave spontaneously. Like predatory African lions, they prey on victims whose body language marks them as easy targets. Both kinds of predator choose victims who they believe won't fight back. Police officers suggest that we humans walk purposely and confidently, with shoulders back, head up, and a destination in mind. This is sound advice. Human beings are primates, and primates are always on the lookout for signs of dominance and submission—of physical strength or physical weakness.

Throughout the world, bowls, baskets, and personal carry bags are considered "women's property." Since a woman's purse sends a message of fragility—as it blatantly announces, "My wallet's inside"—either do not carry a purse or cradle it snugly in front with your dominant hand. The purse strap should look forbiddingly thick to deter casual purse snatchers. Women, avoid wearing showy jewelry or carrying colorful purses that beckon from a distance.

A PREDATORY THREESOME

While shopping in Washington, D.C., my wife was surprised when two young men, one on each side, began walking beside her. They made friendly, bantering chatter as they matched her stride, step for step, on the crowded sidewalk. Remembering the basket purse she'd slung over her right shoulder, she looked back and saw a third man about to reach inside. Two to preoccupy, one to grasp from behind. My wife swung her purse in front, and the trio melted away in the crowd.

Men should know that street thieves sometimes use neckties as convenient nooses to dominate, demean, and control the victims they rob. As you walk a mean street, take off your tie. If you must travel on a vacant city sidewalk, keep clear of concealed doorways and alley entrances from whence thieves can pounce unseen. Watch for predators one block ahead at a time, and cross to the street's safe side to discourage opportunistic grasping. Remember that most street thefts are unplanned and impulsive. Thieves are subject to the whims of their grasping reflex.

APPROACHED FROM BEHIND

While murderers usually know their victims, thieves take from strangers. Street thieves may come at you from any direction, at any time of day or night. In a typical theft scenario, you are alone on foot in unfamiliar territory. You're in a parking lot at night in a phone booth. A car with three young men brakes, turns into the lot, and circles your booth. They seem to be staring at you. You see the whiteness of predatory eyes. A man yells, "Give me your wallet!"

You walk down a deserted city street at 9:00 a.m. A man on a rusty bicycle pedals toward you. He stares at your face from a distance. Coming closer, you see the prominent whites of his eyes, then a gun, as you hear the familiar demand, "Give me your wallet!" When you are alone on the street, beware of an approaching stranger's unfamiliar face. Perhaps a predator comes your way. Cross the street, take the secure route, duck into a store. If the face feels predatory, it likely is.

As you periodically monitor your surroundings, don't forget to check your mental "rearview mirror." Many street thieves approach from behind:

- On April 8, 2000, at 12:40 a.m., a twenty-five-year-old San Francisco man was approached from behind by two men in their twenties (Perillo 2000). The victim opened his wallet and gave up his money. When one of the thieves grabbed for the emptied wallet, the owner reflexively pulled it away and was struck on the head with a handgun.

- On April 9, 2000, at 2:00 p.m., a fifty-one-year-old San Francisco woman was walking when she felt someone behind her pull at her shoulder bag. Turning around, she saw a twenty-year-old man grabbing her purse. The woman struggled with the man, and both fell to the ground. She grabbed his tennis shoe and twisted it off his foot. He grabbed her purse away and fled to a waiting car (Perillo 2000).
- On September 5, 2005, at 1:15 a.m., a University of Rochester male undergraduate returning from an off-campus party was approached from behind by a robber who pressed what felt like a gun into his back as the victim talked on his cell phone. The assailant demanded money and stole the student's phone (Anonymous 2005b).
- On December 21, 2005, at 5:50 p.m., a University of Rochester female undergraduate walking on a sidewalk was approached from behind by a lone male, who grabbed her handbag. He escaped by jumping over a chain-link fence (Anonymous 2005b).

Regularly checking your "rearview mirror" deprives thieves who would approach from behind of the surprise element they sometimes depend on. Robbing a person from the front is fundamentally different from robbing a vending machine or a vacated home. Street thieves who are unable or unwilling to face you directly may cunningly prowl from behind.

BAD NEIGHBOR SIGNS

Treat strangers approaching your home as you would those approaching your body. Both may be afflicted with GHS—grasping hands syndrome. GHS sufferers are constantly in search of something easy to pinch, hook, lift, or grab with their hands.

At home, be wary of strangers on your porch. Police blotters are replete with cases of thieves who rob upon entering—or who punch first and ask questions later. On January 22, 2006, in Spokane, Washington, a resident answered a 7 p.m. knock at his apartment's front door. A masked man with a shotgun, accompanied by two female accomplices, burst in and stole his girlfriend's purse. On January 15, 2007, after politely knocking on the front door, two armed men burst into a couple's Orange County, Florida, home and demanded money and jewels. On February 2, 2007, a forty-three-year-old Warren, Ohio, man answered a knock at his front door. Two men burst in, threatened him with a knife, and stole his house keys, car keys, and cell phone.

More than a century before these incidents, Bernard Picker of Delphos, Ohio, opened his front door to three masked thieves. As the January 1, 1880, edition of the *Delphos Herald* reported, "A knock at the door was answered by the old man, who was immediately felled to the floor by a heavy blow across the eyes."

Each of these crimes was preventable. While you are vulnerable on the street, your home provides a physical barrier—until you open the front door. Before opening, check the outside entryway for potential danger signs. Be leery of strange men who could work as a team, of unfamiliar women who could front for hidden men, and of men carrying anything that could be used as a weapon. If their body language seems abnormally tense or anxious, it's because they've arrived on your porch fully primed for action. You will see adrenaline-charged demeanor, men standing taller, moving faster, showing tense hand gestures. That they lean forward and crowd your doorway telegraphs eagerness to come in. They poise to spring forward should you barely crack open the door.

"Knock-knock" theft happens on a routine basis. To guard against sneak attack, use the color code devised by Colonel Jeff

Cooper for military and police personnel (Cooper 1989). In Code White, you are unaware of your surroundings. (Thieves like it best when victims are blissfully unaware.) In Code Yellow, you are alert to danger on all sides of your home, front and back. In Code Orange, you sense clear and present danger from a specific knock or doorbell ring. Since robbery is always possible, mentally prepare by checking your outside entry. In Cooper's final stage, Code Red, theft is under way—you missed your chance to stand clear. But if you stay in a relaxed-alert frame of mind, this is unlikely. With awareness, you avoid opening a door to danger. As Cooper advises, "If you see a dangerous snake, stay out of his reach."

Be suspicious should an unmarked van pull up to your vacationing neighbor's home. A man in work clothes emerges with an official-looking clipboard. In broad daylight, he will walk to the front door, knock, and ring the bell. Note how he tests the doorknob to see if it's unlocked. If it opens, in he goes, and he exits with items concealed in his "toolbox." If the door's locked, he casually turns and walks around the house, testing for unlocked side doors, open windows, or air conditioners to push in. Get the van's license number and call police.

A U.S. prison poll reveals that the first place burglars look for cash, jewelry, and other valuables is the master bedroom. They forage through pockets, search beneath beds, and feel under mattresses, throw pillows, and rugs. When drapes are open and lights are on, thieves wait to see if anyone walks by a window. A potential welcome sign for house thieves is seeing no car in the driveway. Thieves like to see homes hidden by bushes and trees. Thick foliage not only hides house thieves, but also provides a staging area for stolen goods waiting to be stashed in vehicles' trunks.

"MY EYES WOULD LIGHT UP"

For a firsthand look at house thieves in action, let's ride along with Junior Kripplebauer, leader of the notorious K&A gang from Philadelphia, as he and three colleagues burglarize a home in Texas (Hornblum 2005). They fly in from Philadelphia, rent two midsize cars, and drive to an affluent suburban neighborhood in Houston. One vehicle is strategically parked for use as a "drop car" for the objects they will steal. In the second vehicle, the four-some rides around in search of neighborhood signals telling which houses to hit.

What signals do K&A gang members look for? Homes with expensive, well-tended shrubbery and manicured lawns stand out as signs. Homes near private country clubs and Jewish synagogues stand out as well. The K&A gang prefers homes owned by Jewish victims who are more likely to keep cash and valuables inside the house rather than stored offsite in banks and safe-deposit boxes.

A coveted signal is the mezuzah. A mezuzah is a small con-tainer of biblical verses on parchment affixed to door frames in accordance with Jewish law. For house thieves, seeing a mezuzah on a front door is a sign that riches may be found in the house-hold. As K&A gang member Johnny Boggs reflected, "My eyes would light up and my heart would beat a little faster when I went up to the house to see if anybody was home and saw that mezuzah on the door" (Hornblum 2005).

Our vehicle stops in front of the targeted home. A well-dressed man in an expensive suit and tie, who is carrying a brief-case, gets out and strolls to the front door. From visual cues, he could be the homeowner's business partner. The man knocks, and rings the doorbell. If no one answers, he walks around back look-ing for occupancy clues. Seeing no sign of anyone inside or out, he returns to the front door and gives colleagues the thumbs-up sign. Two expensively dressed partners get out, and then the third drives away.

Rather than pick the lock to get inside, one K&A man breaks out his trusty three-foot-long number 9714 screwdriver and pries open the front door. The men fan out inside and look around, going through chests of drawers and jewelry boxes. They home in on the treasure-trove master bedroom. Cash is almost always found in the master bedroom. As one thief remarked, "They [the victims] love to be near their money" (Hornblum 2005).

The group is in and out in fifteen minutes. The car returns, and they lock their take in the trunk. Fifteen minutes to steal a valuable coin collection, silver goblets, a Rolex watch, and fine jewelry. Then they're off to burglarize three more Houston houses before flying back to their Philadelphia home base. Police, as usual, are mystified. Tonight has been the usual success story.

The infamous K&A gang, who always dressed smartly and never carried guns, robbed homes from Philadelphia to Houston to Miami from the 1950s through the 1970s.

Crime signals that led to the capture of one K&A crew came from reports of witnesses seeing four unfamiliar, well-dressed men driving together through expensive suburban neighborhoods in Pennsylvania. In July 1959, state police arrested that K&A crew in a Williamsport motel, where they found burglary tools, a coin collection, expensive jewelry, and cash. Louis "Junior" Kripplebauer, leader of the K&A crew in Houston, Texas, was finally caught and served time in Pennsylvania's Graterford Prison.

The stories you have read in this chapter are true. Each tells of a person or persons who steal others' property by using their hands to take ownership. To catch a thief, watch for suspicious signs—especially hand movements—to learn if someone may be planning to pilfer your precious stuff:

- A hand testing a doorknob to see if it's unlocked
- A well-dressed stranger with a carry bag casing your condo
- Someone "just like you and me" straining to open a locked door
- Someone on the street who notices you and monitors your presence
- A suspicious young man following close behind
- A "workman" with a clipboard prowling your backyard
- Anyone in your neighborhood carrying a three-foot-long screwdriver

CONCLUSION

ON DECEMBER 12, 2001, something suspicious caught Kenneth Evans's eye. Evans noticed someone he thought was a homeless bag lady shopping in his Beverly Hills store. Her presence within seemed unusual, uncommon, and perceptibly abnormal. While many homeless women frequent Beverly Hills sidewalks, few shop at the swanky Saks Fifth Avenue on Wilshire Boulevard.

On the autumn Wednesday in question, Ken Evans, Saks's security manager, was alerted to a likely theft in progress. As he viewed the disheveled woman's odd-lot bags on his closed-circuit TV—she carried two large shopping bags, a garment bag, and a tote bag—and watched her physical movements through the store as she picked up not fistfuls but armloads of designer clothing and accessories, he sensed something was wrong. In still shots from the security video, the mystery shopper appears to be caught in a final, desperate act of object fancy. Like the proverbial monkey who couldn't dislodge his hand from the cookie jar, so tight was his grasp on cookies inside, the cache of clothing she grasped in her hands and arms threatened to bury her.

Suspicion grew as Evans saw her put on a hat, with its price tag still attached, and enter a changing room—only to emerge with the hat minus its dangling tag. As every security officer knows, shoplifters tend to look at other people rather than at merchandise, and keep returning to the same store area until it's safe to steal. Moreover, shoplifters often appear nervous, and gaze from side to side as they handle items, without actually looking at what they hold. For Ms. Bag Lady, the maxim "Hands do the taking—eyes do the stealing" was true.

She held copious amounts of clothing, but her eyes gazed away.

Ken Evans watched his security screen and assigned fellow Saks employee Colleen Rainey to monitor the shopper of interest. As Rainey peeped through the slats of the young woman's dressing-room door, the robbery plot thickened. Rainey reportedly saw the bag lady kneel on the floor, pull orange-handled scissors from her shoulder bag, and cut the electronic sensor tags off two designer purses. Then she watched her put both purses, along with socks and a hair bow, into another bag.

As the lady continued her ninety-minute shopping spree and roamed the department store's upper two floors, basement-operated surveillance cameras recorded her bags curiously ballooning in size. She was filmed entering dressing rooms on the second and third floors, remaining inside (and off camera) for as long as fifteen minutes at a time, and then exiting with fuller bags. Once, when she lost her balance and dropped the growing load of pilfered goods, Evans spied the hat she'd tried on earlier, showing in the woman's red Saks Fifth Avenue bag.

Acting on the crime signals they saw inside, security guards detained the suspect as she left the department store and escorted her back into the store. The purported bag lady was none other than two-time Oscar nominee and Hollywood actress Winona Ryder, of *Edward Scissorhands* fame. After seeking guidance from Saks's headquarters, security called Beverly Hills police who arrested Ryder, age thirty, at seven that evening. She was booked on charges of felony grand theft, and released on $20,000 bail around eleven thirty that night.

Crime signals had spoken on that December 12, and their meaning rang true. Police found more than $5,000 worth of unpaid merchandise in her bags, including a $760 Marc Jacobs top, $80 cashmere socks, and a $1,600 Gucci dress. On November 6, 2002, after her trial by jury, Winona Ryder was convicted of stealing $5,560 in clothing and accessories from Saks. She was sentenced to three years of probation, ordered to pay Saks for the items she'd taken, and fined $2,700.

Had it not been for ten crime signals—(1) Winona Ryder's anomalous carry bags; (2) her concealment of items within; (3) holding merchandise physically close to her body instead of leaving it with salespeople as she shopped; (4) the abnormal time spent in dressing rooms; (5) the extended stay in the store itself; (6) her arms-fully-loaded show of "object fancy"; (7) the chronically disappearing price tags; (8) her odd kneeling posture on the fitting-room floor; (9) the cutting of sensor tags from handbags with scissors; and (10) her visibly swollen bags—the perpetrator might have gone undetected. Since the likely prognosis for thieves is continuation of illegal grasping until capture, the good lesson for Winona is that capture came sooner rather than later in life. Though she showed little emotion at trial, and no remorse after her conviction—which was never appealed—we trust her criminal days are over for good.

Crime Signals concludes with the body language of thieves because, at base, all criminals engage in theft. Deceivers withhold the truth, predators abduct children, and street gangs rob money—as well as the lives of the youth who join them. Murderers take life; terrorists, peace; and con men, trust. Corporate crooks steal pensions, drugs steal sanity, and stalkers steal peace of mind. Each criminal takes, and gives nothing back in return.

Crime—whether violent, conniving, or petty—is almost never completely unpredictable. Nonverbal signs betray criminals throughout their misdeeds. As we've seen, crime signals are best decoded prior to unlawful acts. Confrontational body language and glaring eyes tipped an alert immigration officer to stop Mohamed al-Kahtani—9/11's "twentieth hijacker"—from possibly helping to blow up the White House. Ahmed Ressam's nervous, sweaty appearance helped an observant customs officer stop the Millennium Bomber's plot to blow up an alcove at Los Angeles International Airport. Zacarias Moussaoui's secretive, standoffish, deceptive, uncooperative, and hotheaded demeanor at flight school led to his capture, and a confession to his role in al Qaeda's plot to crash jetliners into U.S. landmarks.

Equally telling signals, even if they do not actually stop crime, aid in the prosecution of criminal offenders. Winona Ryder's suspicious body language led to her arrest and conviction for shoplifting. Brad Jackson's conspicuous shoulder shrugs on the witness stand cast doubt on his statements about the cause of death of his young daughter, Valiree. Scott Peterson's indifferent, unemotional body language in court paved the way for his death sentence.

The most unfortunate signals are those that are sent and received but are somehow unheeded before tragedy occurs. Kristin Lardner saw, heard, and felt a medley of serious warning signs before boyfriend Michael Cartier shot her from behind. Nicole Simpson saw enraged facial expressions; heard virulent, screaming voice tones; and felt terribly strong hands grip her before her death by stabbing. Throughout this book we've dealt with people whose behavior has been characterized as "creepy." Something creepy produces palpable sensations of unease, apprehension, and fear. Creepy, in short, is the ultimate crime signal.

We have examined and identified the body language of a number of perpetrators throughout this book. These are the nonverbal warning signs that can help you protect yourself, your loved ones, and your property from harm. May the knowledge and insights you gain from watching crime signals keep you safely out of harm's way.

BIBLIOGRAPHY

Alford, Richard (1996). "Adornment." In David Levinson and Melvin Ember (eds.), *Encyclopedia of Cultural Anthropology* (New York: Henry Holt), pp. 7–9.

Andermann, Frederick, and Eva Andermann (1992). "Startle Epilepsy." In Anthony B. Joseph and Robert R. Young (eds.), *Movement Disorders in Neurology and Neuropsychiatry* (Cambridge, Mass.: Blackwell Scientific Publications), ch. 66, pp. 498–500.

Anonymous (1838). "Opium Eating." *Boston Medical and Surgical Journal*, vol. 18 (March 28), pp. 128–29.

Anonymous (1988). *Narcotics Anonymous*, 5th ed. (Chatsworth, Calif.: Narcotics Anonymous World Services).

Anonymous (1998). "Admitting Co-Respondent's Redacted Confession Was Error but Harmless." San Antonio Court of Appeals Judgment (December 30; Texas Juvenile Probation Commission Web document, www.tjpc.state.tx.us).

Anonymous (2000a). "Amygdala Responds Differently When Individuals View Racially Disparate Faces." *Reuters Health* (September 11; a report of findings published in *NeuroReport*, vol. 11 [August 3, 2000], pp. 2351–55).

Anonymous (2000b). *State of Tennessee v. Derrick M. Vernon et al.* Court of Criminal Appeals of Tennessee at Jackson (no. W1998-00612-CCA-R3-CD—decided April 25, 2000).

Anonymous (2001). "Something's Wrong." *U.S. Customs Today* (December).

Anonymous (2002). "Handy Andy." *The Guardian* (November 5; www .guardian.co.uk).

Anonymous (2003a). *Terrorist Hunter* (New York: HarperCollins).

Anonymous (2003b). "U.S. Says No Early Trial for Saddam." BBC News (December 16; news.bbc.co.uk).

Anonymous (2004). "Saddam's 'Defeated' Body Language." BBC News (July 1; news.bbc.co.uk).

Anonymous (2005a). "Father Guilty of Raping Daughters, Holding Family Hostage." *St. Petersburg Times (Fl.)* Associated Press; February 20; http://sptimes.com.

Anonymous (2005b). "Safety Bulletin (Robbery—Main St. Between Swan St. and Gibbs St.)." *University of Rochester Safety Bulletin* (December 22; security.rochester.edu).

Anonymous (2006a). "FBI Seeks Help in Catching 'Gentleman Bandit.'" cbs2chicago.com (April 20; copyright 2006 by *Chicago Sun-Times*).

Anonymous (2006b). "The Man Who Conned Nine Women into Marriage." *The Oprah Winfrey Show* (February 13; www.oprah.com).

Anonymous (2007). "Fla.'s Unwanted Big Business." *Lakeland (Fl.) Ledger* (January 30; www.theledger.com).

Bach, Ashley (2005). "Pickpockets Target Older Women: Team Struck 4 Times." *Seattle Times* (December 22; www.seattletimes.com).

Baker, Leigh (2002). *Protecting Your Children from Sexual Predators* (New York: St. Martin's Press).

Beata, C. A. (2001). "Diagnosis and Treatment of Aggression in Dogs and Cats." In K. A. Houpt (ed.), *Recent Advances in Companion Animal Behavior Problems* (Ithaca, N.Y.: International Veterinary Information Service, www .ivis.org).

Bell, Rachel (2006). "Ted Bundy." Court TV Crime Library (www.crime library.com).

Benecke, Mark (2005). *Murderous Methods: Using Forensic Science to Solve Lethal Crimes* (New York: Columbia University Press).

Blum, Miriam D. (1988). *The Silent Speech of Politicians* (San Diego: Brenner Information Group).

Blurton Jones, N. G. (1967). "An Ethological Study of Some Aspects of Social Behaviour of Children in Nursery School." In Desmond Morris (ed.), *Primate Ethology* (Chicago: Aldine), pp. 347–68.

Borger, Julian (2006). "Gunned Down: The Teenager Who Dared to Walk Across His Neighbour's Prized Lawn." *The Guardian* (March 22; www.guardian.co.uk).

Brown, Peter H., and Pat H. Broeske (1996). *Howard Hughes: The Untold Story* (New York: Dutton).

Bugliosi, Vincent, with Curt Gentry (1974). *Helter Skelter: The True Story of the Manson Murders* (New York: W. W. Norton).

Bugliosi, Vincent (1996). *Outrage: The Five Reasons Why O. J. Simpson Got Away with Murder* (New York: W. W. Norton).

Burge, Kathleen (2002). "Law Notes Regret on Wording." *Boston Globe* (August 3; www.boston.com/globe).

Burrough, Bryan (2004). *Public Enemies: America's Greatest Crime Wave and the Birth of the FBI, 1933–34* (New York: Penguin Press).

Butler, Daniel, Alan Ray, and Leland Gregory (2000). *America's Dumbest Criminals* (New York: Random House).

Byron, Christopher (2002). *Martha Inc.: The Incredible Story of Martha Stewart Living Omnimedia* (New York: John Wiley & Sons).

CBS (2004). Nick Flint's Comment on Scott Peterson's Voice, *48 Hours Mystery* (June 2).

Cheesman, Clive, and Jonathan Williams (2000). *Rebels, Pretenders, and Imposters* (New York: St. Martin's Press).

Chelminski, Rudolph (1999). "Secret Soldier." *Reader's Digest* (April; excerpt of Chelminski's book *Secret Soldier*), pp. 200–1.

Clouse, Thomas (2005). "Youth Pastor Faces Sex Allegations." *Spokane (Wash.) Spokesman-Review*, Spokane (December 20; www.spokesman-review.com).

Cooper, Jeff (1989). *Principles of Personal Defense* (Boulder, Colo.: Paladin Press).

Craig, John (2006a). "Testimony Under Way in Stalking Trial." *Spokane (Wash.) Spokesman-Review* (January 5; www.spokesman-review.com).

Craig, John (2006b). "Judge Finds Spokane Man Guilty of Stalking Woman." *Spokane (Wash.) Spokesman-Review* (January 10; www.spokesman-review.com).

Cramer, James J. (2003). "Bad Boys, Bad Boys." *New York* (October 20; www.nymag.com).

Crompton, Vicki, and Ellen Z. Kessner (2003). *Saving Beauty from the Beast* (New York: Little, Brown).

Cruver, Brian (2002). *Anatomy of Greed: The Unshredded Truth from an Enron Insider* (New York: Carroll & Graf).

Cutler, Brian L., and Steven D. Penrod (1995). *Mistaken Identification: The Eyewitness, Psychology, and the Law* (New York: Cambridge University Press).

Dahlburg, John-Thor (2006). "Abramoff Sentenced in Business Fraud Case." *Los Angeles Times* (March 30; www.latimes.com).

Dahler, Don (2005). "A Real Life 'Catch Me If You Can.'" *20/20* (May 13; www.abcnews.go.com/2020).

Darwin, Charles (1872). *The Expression of the Emotions in Man and Animals*, 3rd ed. (New York: Oxford University Press, 1998).

Dawson, Robert O. (1999). "Questioning That Resulted in Confession Was Not Custodial and Statement Was Voluntary" (1999 Case Summaries; University of Texas School of Law; 99-2-32).

de Becker, Gavin (1997). *The Gift of Fear: Survival Signals* (New York: Little, Brown).

De Leon, Virginia (2004). "Priest Admits to Abusing Boys." *Spokane (Wash.) Spokesman-Review* (September 29; www.spokesman-review.com).

Dodd, Mike, and Hal Bodley (2005). "Steroid Test Nabs First Major Star in Palmeiro." *USA Today* (August 1; www.usatoday.com).

Doria, Kelly, and Joe Menard (2001). "Missouri Threats Surface: Men of Middle Eastern Descent Inquired About Purchasing Planes in Neosho, Local Men Say." *(Springfield (Mo.) News-Leader* (September 27; www.news-leader.com).

Eberly, Tim (2005). "Drug Dealers Erect Shrines to Mexican Folk Hero." *Fresno Bee* (September 30; www.fresnobee.com).

Eibl-Eibesfeldt, Irenaus (1971). "The Expressive Behaviour of the Deaf-and-Blind-Born." In Mario von Cranach and Ian Vine (eds.), *Social Communication and Movement* (European Monographs in Social Psychology 4, New York: Academic Press), pp. 163–94.

Eichenwald, Kurt (2005). *Conspiracy of Fools: A True Story* (New York: Broadway Books).

Elliott, A. Larry, and Richard J. Schroth (2002). *How Companies Lie* (New York: Crown Business).

Feder, George N., with Bob Andelman (2001). "Confessions of an Ex-Jewel Thief." *Weekly Planet* (December 13; www.weeklyplanet.com).

Fenton, Peter (2005). *Eyeing the Flash: The Education of a Carnival Con Artist* (New York: Simon & Schuster).

Ferdinand, Pamela, and Paul Duggan (2002). "In Boston, Driven by Disillusionment." *Washington Post* (October 30; www.washingtonpost.com).

Ferreira, Anton (2006). "Baboons Raiding Houses in South Africa." Reuters Wire Service (May 21; http://articles.news.aol.com).

Ferrer, Gina (2006). "Cocaine Seized Near Border Worth $3.1 Million." *Spokane (Wash.) Spokesman-Review* (March 18; www.spokesman-review.com).

Fetko, Misty (2006). "What Signs Did I Miss?" Article on Web site of the Partnership for a Drug-Free America (May 15; www.drugfree.org).

Fickes, Michael (2003). "Exposing Hostile Intent." *Access Control & Security Systems* (November 12).

Fletcher, Connie (1991). *Pure Cop* (New York: Villard Books).

Flew, Andrew (1979). *A Dictionary of Philosophy* (New York: St. Martin's Press).

Frank, Thomas (2005a). "Airport Security Uses Talk as Tactic." *USA Today* (December 28).

Frank, Thomas (2005b). "Suspects' Body Language Can Blow Their Cover." *USA Today* (December 28; www.usatoday.com).

Frey, Amber (2005). *Witness: For the Prosecution of Scott Peterson* (New York: HarperCollins).

Fuhrman, Mark (2001). *Murder in Spokane* (New York: Cliff Street Books).

Garber, Anne (2003). "Is Martha Stewart Being Unjustly Targeted as an 'Example'?" *Comments by Anne Garber* ("Martha Stewart: A Personal Observation"; http://evaluate.org).

Garrison, Jessica, and Jean Guccione (2006a). "Chronicling Priest's Pattern of Abuse." *Los Angeles Times* (February 8; www.latimes.com).

Garrison, Jessica, and Jean Guccione (2006b). "Wempe Is Convicted on 1 Count" *Los Angeles Times* (February 23; www.latimes.com).

Givens, David B. (1977). "Shoulder Shrugging: A Densely Communicative Expressive Behavior." *Semiotica*, vol. 19, no. 1/2, pp. 13–28.

Givens, David B. (2003). *The Nonverbal Dictionary of Gestures, Signs, and Body Language Cues* (Spokane, Wash.: Center for Nonverbal Studies Press).

Givens, David B. (2005). *Love Signals: A Practical Field Guide to the Body Language of Courtship* (New York: St. Martin's Press).

Glionna, John (2007). " 'Maltese Falcon' Replica Stolen from S.F. Restaurant." *Spokane (Wash.) Spokesman-Review* (February 14; www.spokesman-review.com; from *Los Angeles Times*).

Global Deception Research Team (2006). "A World of Lies." *Journal of Cross-Cultural Psychology*, vol. 37, no. 1, pp. 60–74.

Grimaldi, James V. (2005). "Abramoff Indicted in Casino Boat Purchase." *Washington Post* (August 12; www.washingtonpost.com).

Guccione, Jean (2006a). "Victim Testifies at Priest's Trial" *Los Angeles Times* (January 24; www.latimes.com).

Guccione, Jean (2006b). "Accuser Says He Hid Abuse by Priest" *Los Angeles Times* (January 31; www.latimes.com).

Hall, Elizabeth (1974). "Ethology's Warning: A Conversation with Niko Tinbergen." *Psychology Today*, vol. 7 (March), p. 66.

Hammett, Dashiell (1930). *The Maltese Falcon*. In *The Novels of Dashiell Hammett* (New York: Alfred A. Knopf, 1965), pp. 293–440.

Hazelwood, Robert R., and Janet Warren (1990). "The Criminal Behavior of the Serial Rapist." *FBI Law Enforcement Bulletin* (February), pp. 11–16.

Hewitt, Bill, Lyndon Stambler, Ron Arias, Vickie Bane, Johnny Dodd, Champ Clark, and Frank Swertlow (2004). "Can He Escape His Lies?" *People* (October 1; www.people.com), pp. 66–71.

Hirschkorn, Phil (2006). "Moussaoui Was a Flight School Washout" *CNN* (March 9; www.cnn.com).

Hoffman, Dennis E. (1993). *Scarface Al and the Crime Crusaders* (Carbondale: Southern Illinois University Press).

Hopson, Janet (1980). "Growl, Bark, Whine & Hiss: Deciphering the Common Elements of Animal Language." *Science*, vol. 80 (May–June), pp. 81–84.

Horan, Isabelle, and Diana Cheng (2001). "Enhanced Surveillance for Pregnancy-Associated Mortality, Maryland 1993–1998." *Journal of the American Medical Association*, vol. 285, no. 11, pp. 1455–59.

Hornblum, Allen M. (2005). "Road Companies, Brutes and Safecrackers." *Philadelphia City Paper* (May 26–June 1; www.citypaper.net).

Innes, Brian (2005). *Fakes and Forgeries* (London: Amber Books).

Jackman, Ian (ed.) (2003). *Con Men* (New York: Simon & Schuster).

Johnson, Gene (2001). "Ressam's '99 Arrest Proved a 'Watershed Event.'" *Spokane (Wash.) Spokesman-Review* (December 9; www.spokesman-review.com).

Johnson, Lowell (2005). "Confessions of a Convicted Vending Burglar." *Automatic Merchandiser* (February 28; www.amonline.com).

Karson, Craig N. (1992). "Oculomotor Disorders in Schizophrenia." In Anthony B. Joseph and Robert R. Young (eds.), *Movement Disorders in Neurology and Neuropsychiatry* (Cambridge, Mass.: Blackwell Scientific Publications), ch. 56, pp. 414–21.

Knox, Mike (1995). *Gangsta in the House: Understanding Gang Culture* (Troy, Mich.: Momentum Books).

LaChance, Gerald P. (2005). Personal communication (December 16).

Lane, George, and Virginia Culver (1997). "Who Is Timothy McVeigh?" *Denver Post* (June 14; www.denverpost.com).

Lardner, George, Jr. (1995). *The Stalking of Kristin* (New York: Atlantic Monthly Press).

Lavergne, Gary M. (1997). *A Sniper in the Tower: The Charles Whitman Murders* (Denton: University of North Texas Press).

Lawick-Goodall, Jane van (1968). "The Behaviour of Free-Living Chimpanzees in the Gombe Stream Reserve." *Behavioural Monographs*, vol. 1, pp. 161–311.

Lebor, Adam (1999). "Hungary's Gentleman Bandit" *Salon.com* (August 17; www.salon.com).

Lee, Henry C. (2002). *Cracking Cases: The Science of Solving Crimes* (New York: Prometheus Books).

Levesque, William R. (2003). "Police Can Be Dead Certain, and Wrong." *St. Petersburg Times (Fl.)* (April 6; http://sptimes.com).

Lewis, Diane E. (2005). "Magazine Lists Top 10 'Bosses from Hell.'" *Boston Globe* (June 26; www.boston.com/globe).

Linder, Douglas (2005). "The Impeachment Trial of President Clinton." Famous Trials Homepage (www.law.umkc.edu).

Longrigg, Clare (2004). *No Questions Asked: The Secret Life of Women in the Mob* (New York: Hyperion).

Lynn, Cari (2005). "Avarice." *Johns Hopkins*, vol. 57, no. 4 (September).

MacLeod, Marlee (2005). "Charles Whitman: The Texas Tower Sniper." Court TV Crime Library (www.crimelibrary.com).

MacLin, O. H., and R. S. Malpass (2001). "Racial Categorization of Faces: The Ambiguous Race Face Effect." *Psychology, Public Policy and Law*, vol. 7, no. 1, pp. 98–118.

Marano, Hara Estroff (1995). "Big Bad Bully." *Psychology Today* (September–October; www.psychologytoday.com).

Mason, William (2003). *Confessions of a Master Jewel Thief* (New York: Villard Books).

Maurer, David W. (1940). *The Big Con: The Story of the Confidence Man* (New York: Anchor Books, 1999.

Mauss, Marcel (1925). *The Gift: The Form and Reason for Exchange in Archaic Societies* (New York: W. W. Norton, 1990).

McCormack, Mark H. (1984). *What They Don't Teach You at Harvard Business School: Notes from a Street-Smart Executive* (New York: Bantam Books).

McFarlan, Donald (ed.) (1990). *The Guinness Book of Records 1991* (New York: Facts on File).

Melendez-Perez, Jose E. (2004). "Statement of Jose E. Melendez-Perez to the National Commission on Terrorist Attacks upon the United States." Seventh Public Hearing of the National Commission on Terrorist Attacks upon the United States (www.9-11commission.gov).

Mesulam, M. Marsel (1992). "Brief Speculations on Frontoparietal Interactions and Motor Autonomy." In Anthony B. Joseph and Robert R. Young (eds.), *Movement Disorders in Neurology and Neuropsychiatry* (Cambridge, Mass.: Blackwell Scientific Publications), ch. 89, pp. 696–98.

Michel, Lou, and Dan Herbeck (2001). *American Terrorist: Timothy McVeigh and the Oklahoma City Bombing* (New York: ReganBooks).

Mister, Chloé (2003). "Neighborhood Clubs Block Drug Activity." *Chicago Reporter* (July–August).

Mitani, John C., and David P. Watts (1999). "Demographic Influences on the Hunting Behavior of Chimpanzees." *American Journal of Physical Anthropology*, vol. 109, pp. 439–54.

Morgan, H. Wayne (1981). *Drugs in America: A Social History, 1800–1980* (Syracuse, N.Y.: Syracuse University Press).

Morlin, Bill (2002). "Woman Recalls Surviving Attack by 'Psycho Killer.'" *Spokane (Wash.) Spokesman-Review* (August 14; www.spokesman-review.com).

Morris, Desmond (1994). *Bodytalk: The Meaning of Human Gestures* (New York: Crown Publishers).

Murphy, Bill (2002). "Andrew Fastow: A Study in Contrasts." *Houston Chronicle* (October 2; www.chron.com).

Nash, Jay Robert (1998). *Terrorism in the 20th Century* (New York: M. Evans).

Natarajan, Radha (2003). "Racialized Memory and Reliability: Due Process Applied to Cross-Racialized Eyewitness Identifications." *New York University Law Review*, vol. 78, no. 5 (www.law.nyu.edu/journals/lawreview).

Navarro, Joe (2005). *Hunting Terrorists: A Look at the Psychopathology of Terror* (Springfield, Ill.: Charles C. Thomas).

Navarro, Joe (2006). Personal communication (June 9).

O'Ballance, Edgar (1979). *Language of Violence: The Blood Politics of Terrorism* (San Rafael, Calif.: Presidio Press).

O'Hare, Peggy (2006). "Trial to Put Man Accused of Faking SEAL Status Before the Women Who Say He Duped Them." *Houston Chronicle* (August 7; www.chron.com).

O'Neill, Sean (2002). "Has Thieving Chimp Made a Monkey of the Law?" (November 6; www.telegraph.co.uk).

Oppenheimer, Jerry (1997). *Martha Stewart—Just Desserts* (New York: William Morrow).

Parsons, Jim (2006). "Cooper Sentenced to 15 Years in Jail." *Houstonist* (August 9; www.houstonist.com).

Perillo, Lois (2000). "Police Beat: Look for the Man with the Missing Shoe." *Noe Valley Voice* (May; noevalleyvoice.com).

Reed, Christopher (2004). "Wrong!" *Harvard Magazine* (September–October; www.harvardmagazine.com).

Resnick, Faye D. (1994). *Nicole Brown Simpson: The Diary of a Life Interrupted* (Beverly Hills: Dove Books).

Richmond, Virginia P., James C. McCroskey, and Steven K. Payne (1991). *Nonverbal Behavior in Interpersonal Relations*, 2nd ed. (Englewood Cliffs, N.J.: Prentice Hall).

Rocha, Sharon (2006). *For Laci* (New York: Crown Publishers).

Ryan, Rose (1993). "How I Remember Him." *Boston Review*. (February–March 1996; http://bostonreview.net/BR21.1/ryan.html).

Sachs, Steven L. (1997). *Street Gang Awareness* (Minneapolis: Fairview Press).

Salmons, Stanley (1995). "Muscle." In Peter L. Williams, et al. (eds.), *Gray's Anatomy: The Anatomical Basis of Medicine and Surgery*, 38th ed. (New York: Churchill Livingstone), pp. 737–900.

Salter, Anna C. (2003). *Predators: Pedophiles, Rapists, and Other Sex Offenders* (New York: Basic Books).

Schechter, Harold (1989). *Deviant: The Shocking True Story of Ed Gein, the Original "Psycho"* (New York: Pocket Books).

Schwartz, John (1996). "Voices Say More Than Mere Words: Tone Tells Perception of Others, Study Finds." *Washington Post* (July 22; www.washingtonpost.com).

Seidman, Joel (2006). "Rudy Plea Reveals Abramoff's Worldwide Reach." MSNBC Breaking News (March 31; www.msnbc.com).

Shapiro, Nina (2002). "A Real Charmer: How a Priest Accused of Pedophilia Became a Bellevue Psychotherapist." *Seattle Weekly* (October 18; www.seattleweekly.com).

Smith, Mickenzie, as told to Liza Hamm (2005). "Her Great Escape." *People* (August 15; www.people.com), p. 68.

Smith, Sean (1996). "Tecce Analysis Catches Media Eye." *Boston College Chronicle*, vol. 5, no. 5 (October 31; www.bc.edu).

Snow, Robert L. (1995). *Protecting Your Life, Home, and Property* (New York: Plenum Press).

Soukhanov, Anne E., (ed.) (1992). *The American Heritage Dictionary of the English Language*, 3rd ed. (New York: Houghton Mifflin).

Spitzer, Michelle (2006). "Internet Teen-Sex Sting Nabs Homeland Security Press Aide." *Spokane (Wash.) Spokesman-Review* (April 5; www.spokesman-review.com).

Stewart, James B. (1992). *Den of Thieves* (New York: Simon & Schuster).

Swartz, Mimi, with Sherron Watkins (2003). *Power Failure: The Inside Story of the Collapse of Enron* (New York: Doubleday).

Taibbi, Matt (2006). "Meet Mr. Republican: Jack Abramoff." *Rolling Stone* (March 24; www.rollingstone.com).

Thorndike, Edward L. (1940). *Human Nature and the Social Order* (Cambridge, Mass., MIT Press, 1969).

Vargas, Marjorie Fink (1986). *Louder Than Words: An Introduction to Nonverbal Communication* (Ames: Iowa State University Press).

Vasquez, Joe (2005). "Inside the Interview with Woman Who Found Finger in Chili." CBS5 (San Francisco, Oakland, San Jose, April 11; www.CBS5.com).

Vrij, Aldert, Lucy Akehurst, and Paul Morris (1997). "Individual Differences in Hand Movements During Deception." *Journal of Nonverbal Behavior*, vol. 21, no. 2, pp. 87–102.

Zellner, Wendy, Mike France, and Joseph Weber (2002). "The Man Behind Enron's Deal." *BusinessWeek* online (special report, February 4; www.businessweek.com).